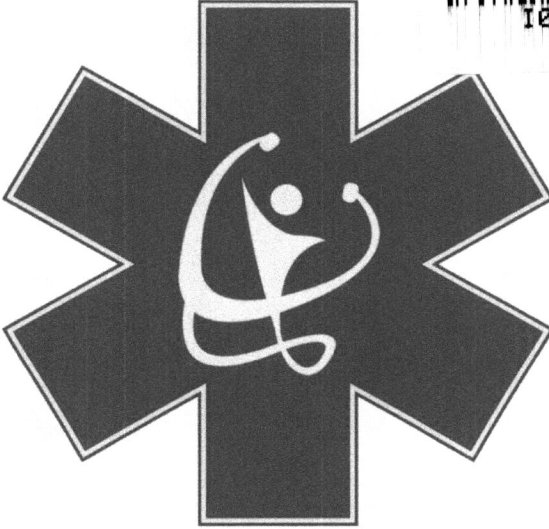

أكاديمية العلوم الصحية
Academy of Health Sciences

Critical Care Nurses' Knowledge and Practices Regarding the Safe Use of Sedatives

Prepared by: Ahmad Mostafa El-Bkkour

Academy of Health Sciences

Critical Care Nurses' Knowledge and Practices Regarding the Safe Use of Sedatives

Thesis

Submitted to the Faculty of Nursing

Alexandria University

In Partial Fulfillment of the Requirements for the Degree

Of Master of Nursing Sciences

In Critical Care and Emergency Nursing

By

Ahmad Mostafa El-Bkkour

Member of the Technical Organization

Faculty of Nursing

Aleppo University

Syrian Arab Republic

2012

SUPERVISORS

Prof. Dr. Azza Hamdi El-Soussi

Professor of Critical Care and Emergency Nursing

Critical Care and Emergency Nursing Department

Faculty of Nursing

University of Alexandria

Dr. Sahar Hossni El-Shenawi

Lecturer of Critical Care and Emergency Nursing

Critical Care and Emergency Nursing Department

Faculty of Nursing

University of Alexandria

Critical Care Nurses' Knowledge and Practices Regarding the Safe Use of Sedatives

Thesis

Presented to the Faculty of Nursing
University of Alexandria
In Partial Fulfillment of the
Requirements for the Degree of

Master of Nursing Sciences

In

Critical Care and Emergency Nursing

By

Ahmad Mostafa El-Bkkour

Examiner's Committee   **Approved**

Prof. Dr. Azza Hamdi El-Soussi   ....

Prof. Dr. Nagwa Mahmoud Al-Kobbia   ....

Prof. Dr. Nagwa Ahmed Reda   ....

Advisors' Committee   **Approved**

Prof. Dr. Azza Hamdi El-Soussi   ....

Dr. Sahar Hossni El-Shenawi   ....

ACKNOWLEDGMENTS

The few words; I wrote here can never and can't adequately express the feelings of gratitude; I have for my supervisors and the persons, who helped me to achieved this work.

I wish to offer my whole-hearted thanks, deepest gratitude and indebtedness to; **Prof. Dr. Azza Hamdi El-Soussi** professor of critical care and emergency nursing, Faculty of Nursing, University of Alexandria, for her continuous advice, tremendous support, valuable guidance, personal attention, sustained encouragement and extreme patience throughout the work of this study. I feel greatly honored to have been working under her supervision.

Words can't adequately express my heartily thanks, profound gratitude, sincere appreciation and indebtedness to **Dr. Sahar Hossni El-Shenawi** lecturer of critical care and emergency nursing, Faculty of Nursing, University of Alexandria, for her expert assistance, honest work, patience, motivation and her willing to devote her time during the various phases of this work to achieve it in the best way. I greatly acknowledge her continuous encouragement and moral support; it was really an honor working under her wonderful supervision.

I would like to express my sincere gratitude, thanks and appreciation to all professors, doctors, staff members and colleagues in the critical care and emergency nursing department for teaching, helping, support and motivating me. I would like to express my great appreciation to all professors and doctors who participated in the jury for the tools.

I would like to express my heartily thanks for the critical care nurses working in casualty ICU & General ICU at Alexandria Main University Hospital for being very helpful during the time of data collection.

My thanks go to Alexandria University and the Faculty of Nursing who helped me in making my dream comes true.

Thanks to my beloved Country......**Syria**

LIST OF ABBREVIATIONS

Abbreviations	Full words
AACN	American Association of Critical Care nurses
BIS	Bispectral index monitor
CBF	Cerebral blood flow
CNS	Central nervous system
D_5W	Dextrose-5%-water
EEG	Electroencephalogram
ETT	Endotracheal tube
GABA	Gamma-Aminobutyric Acid
ICP	Intracranial pressure
ICU	Intensive care unit
IM	Intramuscular
IV	Intravenous
Kcal	Kilocalorie
LOC	Level of consciousness
MAEs	Medication adverse drug events
MASS	Motor Activity Assessment Scale
mL	Milliliters
NaCl	Sodium chloride
RASS	Richmond Agitation-Sedation Scale
RSS	Ramsay Sedation Scale
SAS	Sedation Agitation Scale

Chapter 1

INTRODUCTION

Introduction

Sedation is an essential component of the management of critically ill patients. It is estimated that 90% of critically ill patients require sedation and analgesia for at least part of their stay in an intensive care unit (ICU). Patients in the ICU are in a foreign environment; usually confined to bed, often are mechanically ventilated and attached to equipment via tubes. Moreover, their family members are not continuously available for comfort. They experience pain, fear and loss of control. Furthermore, the significant noise from personnel and medical equipment can increase anxiety and disrupt their normal sleep patterns. The loss of normal circadian rhythms, the disruption of normal sleep patterns and the awareness of discomfort all contribute to patients anxiety and promote the development of psychological stress [1, 2].

Providing adequate sedation is an important but often poorly managed component of critical care treatment and support. This aspect of critical care management is often lost in the myriad of hemodynamic, respiratory and metabolic derangements that are frequently encountered and often overwhelm the practitioner [3].

Sedative drugs are administered primarily to improve comfort, minimize physical and psychological stress, induce amnesia, facilitate mechanical ventilation, facilitate patient-ventilator synchrony, improve tolerance of routine ICU procedures, promote sleep, prevent self harm, promote hemodynamic stability and reduce intracranial pressure [4-6].

The appropriate target level of sedation is calm patients that can be easily aroused with maintenance of the normal sleep-wake cycle. Monitoring sedation level is very important in determining patient outcomes as both undersedation and oversedation of critically ill patients are undesirable and are associated with complications and both have an obvious effect on morbidity and mortality. A study conducted by Kaplan and Bailey [7] who found that 15.4% of ICU patients were under-sedated in the course of their care, while 30.6% were properly sedated. Interestingly, 54% of these patients were over sedated. To avoid under-or over sedation, the use of sedation protocol and sedation scoring system to regularly assess and document sedation level, have been recommended. The establishment of endpoints of sedation has been demonstrated to improve clinical practice of sedation [4, 8-17].

Critical care nurses have a major role in the management of sedation in critically ill patients in collaboration with medical staff to achieve agreed target levels of sedation. Nurses play a key role in selecting the most appropriate and safest sedative agent because they may be best able to monitor the efficacy of the chosen sedative and to observe patients for potential adverse events and complications [18, 19].

Ensuring safe and effective administration of medications to patients is a fundamental responsibility of the nurse. An understanding of the basic concepts of administering drugs is critical if nurses are to perform this task safely and accurately. Administering medications involves more than just the technical task. Therefore; nurses must have factual knowledge of each drug given, the reasons for use of the drug, the drug's general action, the more common adverse reactions associated with the drug, special precautions in administration (if any), and the normal dose ranges [20].

There is a need to document what is done daily in ICUs because there may be a substantial gap between the current recommendations and clinical practices. Therefore, this study is carried out in order to identify critical care nurses' knowledge and practices regarding the safe use of sedatives and to reflect what is really done regarding sedation practices in the critical care units of the Main University Hospital of Alexandria.

Chapter II

Review of Literature

Literature review

Critically ill patients are a heterogeneous group with different underlying co morbid conditions, severity of illness, monitoring needs and requirements for life support. They are often scared, disorientated, isolated and cannot communicate easily how they feel and what they need to feel better. They are surrounded by plastic tubes, ventilators, bright light and strange noises. They have also lost intimate contact with their families or loved ones, are surrounded by strangers and are no longer in control. Therefore, providing comfort to these patients continues to be complex [21].

Sedation management forms an integral component of the care of critically ill patients. Carrasc et al [22], state that in Australia 70% of intensive care unit patients require sedation at least one time during their hospital stay. In this regard, in England 76% of patients who undergo mechanical ventilation need sedation and this rate is 60% in Italy [23, 24]. In Egypt, Ba-alwi A (2008) [25] found that about the half of critically ill patients were sedated.

Sedative overview

The word 'sedate' is derived from the Latin word sedare, which means 'to calm'. It is a non-specific word used to explain the action of an agent as it moves patients toward a calm relaxed state. Sedatives are drugs that calm patients down, easing agitation and permitting sleep. It generally works by modulating signals within the central nervous system. In the past, sedative agents were generally used to keep patients motionless and to reduce memory of their experience in the ICU. However, recognition that heavy sedation may increase mortality and morbidity has led to a new model in which the emphasis is on maximizing the comfort of these patients while they remain interactive, oriented, and able to follow instructions [26, 27].

It is important to recognize that the sedation goal is a two-tiered goal. The primary goal is the "why" goal, or the reason for sedation. The secondary goal is the "how much" goal or the desired degree of sedation. The "why" goal, drives the decision to determine the individualized need for sedation. While, the "how much" goal ensures the individualized need for sedation. In intensive care settings, there are a variety of reasons to chemically sedate patients. However, three of the primary indications for sedation are: injury prevention, facilitation of medical goals and humanitarian goals [28, 29].

The first reason for sedation is that patients, if left without adequate sedation, may cause injury to themselves or others. This may include removal of medically necessary monitoring or support devices as well as causing injury to the staff members caring for them while they are in a state of delirium. The brain injured patients may, for instance, be cognitively impaired and incapable of understanding the necessity of the many tubes and purposefully attempt to remove these tubes. Another example of injury to self is patients who bite down on endotracheal tubes; that results in the risk of eventually biting the tubing in half, and the more immediate threat of injury by occluding the only patent airway available for lung ventilation. Adequate sedation will impair the ability to harm themselves, or others, by decreasing the ability to generate physical actions. In addition, promoting synchronized breathing with the ventilator [29-31].

The second reason for sedating a patient is to facilitate the medical goals set for patients. This includes goals such as maintaining hemodynamic goals, decreasing excess oxygen consumption, increasing ventilatory compliance, controlling intracranial pressure, treating patients with status epilepticus, treating sleep disorders and delirium [4, 29, 31-34].

The third reason for sedating patients is for humanitarian intentions. In all patients receiving neuromuscular blockade complete and deep sedation is mandatory to avoid the mental distress associated with total body paralysis. Adequate sedation of critically ill patients also becomes paramount when an individual is inflicted with a barrage of noxious stimuli and invasive procedures such as the insertion of intracranial pressure (ICP) monitoring devices or placement of medically necessary catheters and monitoring devices. Adequate sedation also results in a degree of induced amnesia for the events associated with the intensive care admission thus protecting patients against the long term emotional stress of the acute illness. Although each of these three reasons is valid enough to justify sedation; often the needs may overlap [29, 35, 36].

The sedation goal must be individualized to the need for sedation. If the indication for sedation is one of injury prevention a lighter state of sedation is likely indicated, such that patients are cooperative but still able to communicate with the staff. If the indication for sedation is to facilitate an individual medical goal, the sedation level may need to be somewhat deeper. The most challenging situation involving sedation is the one in which the indication for sedation is for humanitarian needs. It is here seen greatest variability in depth of sedation required in order to provide comfort for a given individual. Sedation for palliative care may range from mild to deep sedation based upon the individual desires of the patient and family. For patients who are chemically paralyzed it is highly undesirable to experience an awakened state, thus most staff prefers to err on the side of a deeper level of sedation. American Society of Anesthesiologists has defined four levels of sedation: minimal sedation, moderate sedation, deep sedation and general anesthesia [28, 37-40].

14

Minimal sedation is defined as a state in which patients respond normally to verbal commands, cognitive function and coordination may be impaired while ventilatory and cardiovascular functions are unaffected. Minimal sedation is used for procedures that require patients to be relaxed but remain responsive such as central line placement, bone marrow aspiration, minor surgical operations and radiologic examinations [40].

Moderate sedation is defined as a state of diminished level of consciousness; arousable by verbal or light tactile stimulus. This state of depressed consciousness is beneficial in procedures that require patients to be immobile for short periods. Procedures that use moderate sedation include chest tube insertion, **temporary pacemaker insertion**, **cardioversion**, **lumbar puncture**, **liver biopsy**, endoscopy, magnetic resonance imaging and various radiological examinations [40, 41].

Deep sedation is a level of depressed consciousness that requires repeated deep tactile stimulation to achieve a purposeful response. Procedures that use deep sedation include airway intubation, patients requiring mechanical ventilation **and** surgeries that incorporate local anesthesia [40].

General anesthesia produces a complete loss of consciousness, requiring mechanical ventilation for airway support as well as medications to support cardiovascular constancy. General anesthesia is used for invasive operations that require complete anesthesia. Analgesics, neuromuscular blockade, and sedative hypnotics are used to induce and maintain sedation [40].

Oversedation versus undersedation

Failure to reach an adequate level of sedation can lead to many sedation complications. Over the last 20 years, research has highlighted the adverse effects that over- or undersedation can have on patient outcomes in the ICU. Therefore, management of sedation in ICU should seek a balance between oversedation with its associated complications and undersedation along with its associated complications [42].

Oversedation is the administration of sedatives at a level greater than the amount of drug required by the individual to achieve the desired effect. Oversedation is common to many ICU settings and more dangerous to the physical wellbeing than under-sedation, as it is associated with dangerous complications and because it may not manifest until well into the recovery period, after the treatment has finished. Oversedation may produce prolonged alteration in consciousness and inability of patients to communicate with health care providers or family members. Furthermore, oversedation can lead to bradycardia, hypotension, respiratory depression, increased period of mechanical ventilation, slow weaning, increased risk of ventilator associated pneumonia and ventilator associated lung injury resulting in increased ICU length of stay, increased diagnostic testing and increased the costs [8, 29, 30, 43, 44].

Undersedation is the administration of sedatives at a level inadequate to meet the sedation goals set by the medical team. Undersedation is less common to the critical care settings than oversedation; the morbidity associated with undersedation can be quite profound. Inadequate sedation can lead to decreased patient safety and increased risk of injury. Compromised patient safety as a result of undersedation is most easily manifest in the example of patients removing intravenous/intra-arterial lines, and unplanned self-extubation. Undersedation may contribute to ventilatory dysynchrony, increased oxygen consumption, delirium, episodes of hemodynamic and intracranial instability and patient movement during procedures [29, 45-49].

Sedative agents in ICU

The ideal sedative has been described as one that works rapidly; provides anxiolysis, sedation, amnesia, or a combination of these; allows quick emergence when stopped; permits easy administration and adjustment of dosage; produces no active metabolites, significant adverse effects or drug-drug interactions and is inexpensive. No drug meets all these criteria. Therefore, clinicians must choose a sedative according to the patient's condition [50, 51].

Sedatives can be divided into four main categories: *benzodiazepines* such as midazolam, diazepam and lorazepam, *barbiturates* such as thiopental, pentobarbital and phenobarbital, *neuroleptic agents* such as haloperidol and *miscellaneous agents* such as propofol, ketamine, clonidine, dexmedetomidine, and isoflurane [34].

Benzodiazepines are central nervous system (CNS) depressants which have sedating, hypnotic and anxiolytic properties, and do not have analgesic properties. They are commonly divided into two broad categories; short and long-acting preparations. The effects of the short acting preparation last for one to three hours while the long acting typically last for six to twelve hours. Clearly, even within the class of benzodiazepines, it is important to select the sedative agent carefully, anticipating how long the patient will be sedated and how long it will take to recover from the sedative state. The major unwanted side effects associated with the benzodiazepines are dose-related respiratory depression and hypotension. If needed, flumazenil (romazicon) is the antidote used to reverse benzodiazepine overdose in symptomatic patients. The most frequently used critical care benzodiazepines are midazolam, diazepam and lorazepam [52-54].

16

Midazolam (dormicum, versed) is recommended for control of acute short-term agitation because of an intravenous onset of action of under 3 minutes. Its short clinical half-life (2-6 hrs) allows the patient to wake up predictably after one-time use. Midazolam also has a nice amnestic effect, which may be ideal for short-term ICU procedures. It is easily titrated and associated with less pain at the injection site. However, continuous use of midazolam has been characterized by prolonged sedative affects, and therefore, it should be used only for short-term continuous infusion. Patients treated with midazolam rarely develop paradoxical reactions characterized by restlessness, agitation, anxiety and sometimes aggressive behaviour [4, 53-57].

Diazepam (neuril, valium) has anticonvulsant properties and produce skeletal muscle relaxation and may be indicated to patients with status epilepticus/uncontrolled seizures. Have an onset of action of 3 to 5 minutes and a half-life of 20 to 50 hours. Diazepam is not recommended for continuous infusion due to precipitation in intravenous (IV) fluids and absorption of diazepam into infusion bags and tubing. IV injection may cause burning and venous irritation [55].

Lorazepam (ativan) is the preferred agent in the ICU for prolonged treatment of anxiety in critically ill patients. **Lorazepam** has an onset of action of 15 to 30 minutes; although, its clinical half-life (10–16 hrs) and it has no active metabolites and wake-up times after continuous infusion with lorazepam are the same or less than midazolam. When using lorazepam by continuous infusion, titrating the intravenous drip up and down does not result in immediate increases nor decreases in blood levels of the drug because of its long half-life [55].

Barbiturates are a sedative-hypnotic that act to increase **gamma-amino butyric acid** (GABA) response in the CNS resulting in a sensation of euphoria and relaxation. There is no analgesia achieved with these medications; therefore, their use is limited to interventions that are not painful. Barbiturates are associated with a high addiction rate and depress neurological function, including the brain stem, which results in depressed electroencephalogram (EEG) activity and seizure cessation [58, 59].

Barbiturates are less commonly used due to their long duration of action, problems with accumulation, narrow therapeutic index and hence potential toxicity. Barbiturates are potent respiratory and cardiovascular depressants. They do not produce muscle relaxation and may paradoxically heighten pain intensity. Furthermore; all barbiturates have a high **propensity** to interact with other drugs which can complicate therapy particularly in critically ill patients who receive multiple drug therapy. It is important to remember that there is no antagonist available for the barbiturates. Any complications that develop should be managed with supportive therapies until the sedative effects are cleared. Thiopental, pentobarbital and phenobarbital **are examples of barbiturates** [58, 60].

17

Thiopental (pentothal) is commonly used in bolus form as an anesthetic induction agent, or for control of seizures or ICP by continuous IV infusion. Thiopental has beneficial effects on ICP by decreasing both cerebral blood flow (CBF) and cerebral metabolic rate. It has a low clearance, thus accumulation is a serious concern, and may lead to myocardial depression and immunosupression [30, 61, 62].

Pentobarbital (nembutal) is classified as a short acting barbiturate; this agent is typically preferable to thiopental when prolonged infusions are anticipated. Pentobarbital infusions have historically been used to reduce refractory intracerebral hypertension, although the hemodynamic and other adverse consequences may have life-threatening consequences [62, 63].

Phenobarbital (luminal) is definitely the long acting drug of the group, with a plasma half-life of up to 140 hrs. **The primary action of phenobarbital is to enhance the inhibitory actions of gamma-aminobutyric acid (GABA) and it is** very effective in the treatment of seizure disorders. Of interest, phenobarbital is the only barbiturate that can be classified as an anticonvulsant drug [62, 63].

Neuroleptic drugs, also called antipsychotic drugs, are commonly used to manage delirium and thought to act by exerting a stabilizing effect on cerebral function, reducing hallucinations, delusions, and unstructured thought patterns. Haloperidol is the most common due to its safer pharmacodynamic profile [30].

Haloperidol (haldol) is still used in some ICUs as a primary sedative. It has no analgesic or amnesic properties and has a long half-life and commonly used for the management of agitated or delirious patients who fail to respond adequately to nonpharmacologic interventions or other sedatives. Patients receiving haloperidol demonstrate indifference to their surrounding environment and may even have cataleptic immobility, making it difficult to perform pain and sedation assessment. The principal concerns with the use of haloperidol are prolongation of the QT-interval and hypotension. Therefore, monitoring the QT interval is mandatory for all patients receiving haloperidol by continuous infusion [4, 34].

Miscellaneous agents: *Propofol (diprivan)* is an intravenous, general anesthetic agent; prescribed only for intubated patients. However, sedative and hypnotic properties can be demonstrated at lower doses. Propofol has a rapid onset and short duration of sedation once discontinued. It is not a reliable amnesic, therefore; it is important to add an opiate such as fentanyl to ensure adequate amnesia. Propofol has been used to sedate neurosurgical patients to reduce elevated intracranial pressure. The rapid awakening from propofol allows interruption of the infusion for neurologic assessment. Propofol may also decrease cerebral blood flow and metabolism.

18

Propofol quickly crosses the blood brain barrier, slows cerebral metabolism, and decreases elevated intracranial pressure [64- 66].

Significant disadvantages of propofol are mainly related to the high lipid content. It comes packaged in a glass container and has the appearance of milk. Propofol is emulsified in a soybean intralipid emulsion that delivers 1.1 kcal /mL as fat. These calories must be taken into account when assessing nutritional intake. Propofol can elevate serum triglyceride levels and has been associated with pancreatitis. The lipid emulsion can also act as a potential medium for bacterial growth. Other adverse effects commonly seen with propofol include bradycardia, hypotension and pain upon peripheral venous injection [65].

Ketamine (ketaset, ketalean) is a short acting sedative-hypnotic-analgesic that induces hypnosis and amnesia; it also acts on opioid binding sites providing analgesia. Ketamine **is useful in patients who require repeated painful procedures such as wound debridement. Ketamine increases intracranial pressure and should be avoided in patients with head injuries or any other conditions that may cause an increase in intracranial pressure** [34, 67].

Clonidine (catapres) is prescribed for patients experiencing withdrawal symptoms. These symptoms may occur after long-term sedation with midazolam and morphine infusions. When attempting to awaken patients, **they** may become agitated and at risk of prematurely removing monitoring equipment or their endotracheal tubes. Clonidine therefore may be useful in 'smoothing out' the period of withdrawal [55, 68].

Dexmedetomidine (precedex) is a highly selective a_2-adrenergic agonist that produces sedation, have both sedative and analgesic properties. It is used as a short-term sedative for less than 24 hours for mechanically ventilated patients. Patients receiving this drug are sedated when undisturbed, but they arouse easily with minimal stimulation, allowing frequent neurologic examinations. Dexmedetomidine is reported to be analgesic sparing in postoperative patients. It causes no respiratory depression, but cardiovascular side effects include bradycardia and hypotension [34, 69, 70].

Isoflurane (forane, terrell) have analgesic, amnestic, and hypnotic properties. Isoflurane has been used in concentrations of up to 0.6% and produces good long term sedation with minimal cardiorespiratory side effects and yet rapid awakening. **The lack of necessary equipment led to limited use of volatile anesthetics as sedative agents in ICUs** [71-73].

Sedatives may be given to a patient intravenously (IV), intramuscularly (IM), orally or by inhalation route. The intravenous route is preferred because it has a fast onset of action and its absorption is more predictable. It is also easier to titrate doses of IV drugs. For intramuscular route; the time of onset or a drug concentration is dependent on blood flow at the site of injection and is unreliable. Similarly, the enteral route is best avoided because the gastrointestinal tract commonly fails in critically ill patients and is also unpredictable [74, 75].

The reasons why inhalational sedation has not gained more widespread acceptance may be of a technical and educational nature. First, critical care ventilators do not allow an easy fitting of vaporizers and there are concerns about excessive agent consumption and environmental contamination which would require a gas scavenging system. Second, there is a little room for an anesthetic machine in critical care units and such machines do not have all the new assisted ventilatory modes used for critical care patients. Finally, from a clinical management perspective, the ICU staff, in general, is not familiar with the pharmacology, physiologic effects, and handling of volatile anesthetics [76].

An intravenous (IV) rout is the most commonly used for administration of sedatives in ICUs. Two ways of IV route are available for sedative drugs; these include intermittent bolus injection and continuous IV infusion. Some sedation strategies favour intermittent intravenous boluses over a continuous infusion [21, 77].

Bolus sedation generally uses less of a sedative, accordingly patients recover more quickly from the effects of the sedative and the costs are lower. Nonetheless these advantages are offset by the reduced comfort of the patient, which in due course may distract the nurses' attention from other equally important patient care issues [78].

In contrast, *continuous IV infusions* provide a more constant level of sedation, which avoids 'peaks and valleys', thus providing better comfort for patients. Continuous IV sedation also frees the nurses' time to address multiple issues. However, continuous infusions also have several disadvantages, they lead to sedatives accumulation in the body over time and as a result patients often become oversedated. Also, withdrawal symptoms (such as tachycardia, hypertension, fever, tachypnea, pupillary dilation, agitation, delirium, seizures) may be seen in patients receiving prolonged infusions of sedatives. Continuous infusion of sedatives also limits the nurse or physician's ability to determine the patient's neurological state and may be troubling to family members who seek cognitive interactions with critically ill patients [21, 27].

To minimize the potential of oversedation with the use of continuous infusions, the concept of daily drug interruption with reintroduction of the infusions at a reduced rate, if necessary, has been explored. Daily interruption of continuous sedative infusions can reduce many of the sedation complications including duration of mechanical ventilation and ICU length of stay. This strategy allows patients to spend some of their ICU time awake and interactive, potentially reducing the amount of sedative given. Sedation protocols may allow the depth of sedation to be decreased without compromising the stated goals of sedation [8, 79-80].

The thought of decreasing or stopping sedatives in critically ill patients who have been agitated may be unsettling. Clinicians may aggressively sedate patients early in their ICU course and then maintain the same level of deep sedation indefinitely. A daily break from sedatives can eliminate the tendency to "lock in" to a high sedative infusion rate that, while appropriate early in ICU care, may be unnecessary on subsequent days. When sedative infusions are decreased or stopped tissue stores can redistribute drug back into the circulation. Interruption of sedative infusions may lead to abrupt awakening and agitation. This must be anticipated by the ICU team to avoid complications such as patient self-extubation. If excessive agitation is noted, sedatives should be resumed [80].

When awakening patients from sedation, for some the ideal may be to reach the brink of consciousness without precipitating excessive agitation. Once objective signs of consciousness are demonstrated, restarting sedatives as needed is reasonable. Restarting the sedative infusion at half of the previous dose also is reasonable. Adjustments from this starting point can be individualized to patient needs [80].

Sedation level determination

Control of the level of sedation of ICU patients is mandatory if the complications associated with over and undersedation are to be avoided. There are a number of subjective and objective measures available to aid in the assessment and adjustment of sedation therapy, to help avoid over- or under-sedation and their consequences, and to manage critically ill patients more precisely [6, 48, 81].

Subjective sedation scales are bedside tools used to determine the level of sedation a patient is exhibiting. They allow for medication titration to achieve a preset sedation goal. Subjective scales rely on examiner interpretation of observed patient behavior. Subjective scales are numerically based; the clinician assesses the patient's response to verbal or tactile stimulus and applies the scales numerical, behavioral correlate. The examinations are performed at a predetermined frequency, usually once an hour and the results are influenced by the patient's sedation level at that exact moment in time. Sedation scales were formulated to improve sedation related complications and improve communication of nurses and physicians as well as decrease ventilatory times, shorten length of stay and lower hospital costs [82, 83].

21

While there are many subjective sedation scales available; few have been appraised with good reliability and validity and none have been chosen as a favorable scale. The four most common subjective scales used in critical care settings are Ramsay Sedation Scale (RSS), Riker Sedation-Agitation Scale (SAS), Motor Activity Assessment Scale (MASS) and Richmond Agitation-Sedation Scale (RASS). These scales are very similar in construction but vary in the descriptions used to assess sedation levels [84, 85].

Ramsay Sedation Scale (RSS), (figure 1), is a single-item tool that allows for three levels of consciousness scoring in patients who are awake and three levels of consciousness scoring in patients who are judged to be asleep. Therefore to use the Ramsay scale the practitioner must first determine if the patient is awake or asleep. If the patient is deemed to be awake they will be given a score of 1, 2, or 3; patients who are asleep will be given a score of 4, 5, or 6 [29].

If an awake score is indicated, the assessor next grades the patient's responsiveness. Awake patients who are responding to stimuli in an agitated manner are scored 1, awake patients who are oriented and respond in a calm and cooperative manner are scored 2, and awake patients who require verbal stimuli to produce a response are scored a 3. If the patient is deemed to be asleep the assessor administers verbal and tactile stimulation. A loud auditory stimulus, such as calling the patient's name, and a glabellar tap (tapping the forehead), are used as stimulus for sleeping patients. Hence, the score for patients who are asleep is based on a brisk (Ramsay = 4), sluggish (Ramsay = 5) or lack of response (Ramsay = 6) to these stimuli. Ramsay values of 1 indicate an inadequate (undersedation) level of sedation, Ramsay values of 2-5 are adequate levels of sedation, and Ramsay values of 6 indicate an excessive (oversedation) level of sedation [29].

Riker Sedation-Agitation Scale (SAS), (figure 2), is a seven-point scale, measures sedation based upon clinical behaviors. SAS **scores a patient's level of consciousness and agitation from a seven item list describing patient behavior.** It has been shown to be reliable and valid in the critically ill adult and has good inter-rater reliability [4].

Motor Activity Assessment Scale (MAAS), (figure 3), is a seven-point scale. It was derived from the SAS for the purpose of being able to evaluate patient behaviors in response to external stimuli. This scale has been shown to have good validity and reliability [82].

Richmond Agitation-Sedation Scale (RASS), (*figure 4*), is a ten-point scale in which positive values are used for agitation and negative values are used for sedation. It was proven to have excellent reliability and validity in comparison with other scales [84].

Ramsay Sedation Scale (RSS)

Score		Response

1	Awake	Patient is anxious and agitated or restless, or both
2		Patient is co-operative, oriented, and tranquil
3		Patient responds to commands only
4	Asleep	Patient exhibits brisk response to light glabellar tap or loud auditory stimulus
5		Patient exhibits a sluggish response to light glabellar tap or loud auditory stimulus
6		Patient exhibits no response

Figure (1) [86]

Riker Sedation-Agitation Scale (SAS)

Score	Term	Descriptor
7	Dangerous agitation	Pulling at endotracheal tube (ETT), trying to remove catheters, climbing over bedrail, striking at staff, trashing side-to-side
6	Very agitated	Does not calm despite frequent verbal reminding of limits, requires physical restraints, biting ETT
5	Agitated	Anxious or mildly agitated, attempting to sit up, calms down to verbal instructions
4	Calm and cooperative	Calm, awakens easily, follows commands
3	Sedated	Difficult to arouse, awakens to verbal stimuli or gentle shaking but drifts off again, follows simple commands
2	Very sedated	Arouses to physical stimuli but does not communicate or follow commands, may move spontaneously
1	Unarousable	Minimal or no response to noxious stimuli, does or communicate or follow

Figure (2) [86]

Motor Activity Assessment Scale (MAAS)

Score	Definition
0	Unresponsive Does not move with noxious stimuli
1	Responsive only to noxious stimuli. Opens eyes or raises eyebrows or turns head toward stimulus or moves limbs with noxious stimuli
2	Responsive to touch or name. Opens eyes or raises eyebrows or turns head toward

	stimulus or moves limbs when touched or name is loudly spoken
3	Calm and cooperative. No external stimulus is required to elicit movement and patient adjusts sheets or clothes purposefully and follows commands
4	Restless and cooperative. No external stimulus is required to elicit movement and patient picks at sheets or tubes or uncovers self and follows commands
5	Agitated. No external stimulus is required to elicit movement and attempts to sit up or moves limbs out of bed and does not consistently follow commands (for example, lies down when asked but soon reverts back to attempts to sit up or move limbs out of bed)
6	Dangerously agitated, uncooperative. No external stimulus is required to elicit movement and patient pulls at tubes or catheters or thrashes side to side or strikes at staff or tries to climb out of bed and does not calm down when asked

Figure (3) [82]

Richmond Agitation Sedation Scale (RASS)

Score	Term	Descriptor
+4	Combative	Overtly combative or violent, immediate danger to staff
+3	Very agitated	Pulls on or removes tubes or catheters or has aggressive behavior toward staff
+2	Agitated	Frequent nonpurposeful movement or patient ventilator dyssynchrony
+1	Restless	Anxious or apprehensive but movements not aggressive or vigorous
0	Alert and calm	
-1	Drowsy	Not fully alert, but has sustained (more than 10 seconds) awakening, with eye contact/eye opening to voice
-2	Light sedation	Briefly (less than 10 seconds) awakens with eye contact to voice
-3	Moderate sedation	Any movement (but no eye contact) to voice
-4	Deep sedation	No response to voice, but any movement to physical stimulation
-5	Unarousable	No response to voice or physical stimulation

Figure (4) [86]

Objective sedation scales are based on physiological measures that are performed on a continuous basis and do not require the assessor to interact with the patient. **Objective testing of a**

patient's level of sedation may be helpful during very deep sedation or when therapeutic neuromuscular blockade masks observable behavior. These scales utilize either vital signs or neurofunction monitors to evaluate sedation levels [4, 83].

Vital signs are a routine component of the ICU assessment. The term vital signs is generally used to describe the set of physiologic measures used for assessing the level of consciousness in a sedated patient. Vital signs include heart rate, blood pressure, respiratory rate, temperature, and most recently, some assessment of the patient's level of pain. In ICU settings vital signs are measured and recorded electronically through monitors attached to the patient. Vital signs are not sensitive markers of sedation and therefore should not be used as the sole source of medication titration [83].

Neurofunction monitors such as electroencephalogram (EEG) monitoring and bispectral index monitor (BIS) are the most commonly used objective scales. EEG monitoring is performed using multiple scalp electrodes that are placed on the skin of the frontal, temporal, parietal, and occipital areas of the cranium. When the waveforms are static and random the patient is awake as they move towards unconsciousness they become more cohesive [83].

Bispectral index monitor (BIS) monitor, (figure 5), is especially helpful for the deeply sedated patient receiving neuromuscular blockade. The BIS uses four sensors that are applied to the skin of the forehead that extent along the temple and above the eye. The BIS monitor displays a number of 0-100 based on the processed EEG signal, a score of 90 to 100 correlates with an awake state, scores in the 70 to 80 with moderate sedation, scores in the 60 to 70 with deep sedation, and scores from the 40 to 60 with general anesthesia [47, 87].

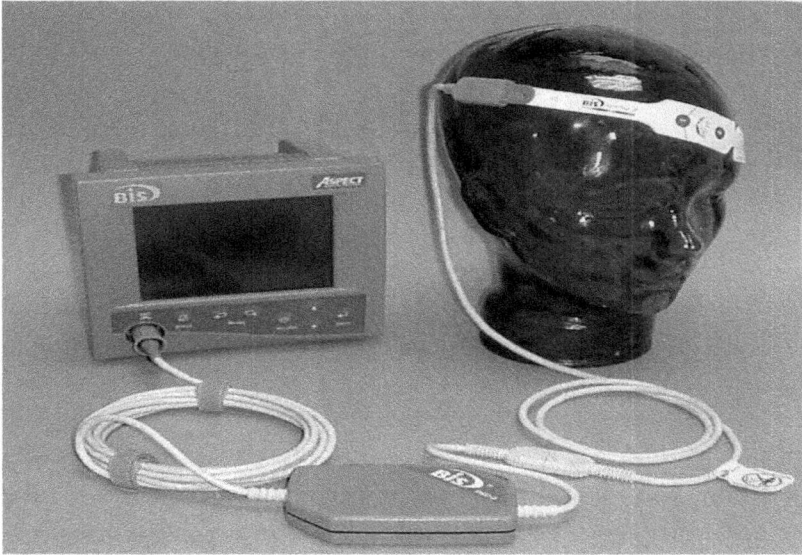

Figure (5) [88]

Safe use of sedatives

An essential component of ensuring quality nursing care in the critical care unit is the maintenance of adequate sedation levels. Critical care nurses have a key role to play in the sedation management practices as they are continuously at the bedside of critically ill patients [21, 89].

Sedative drugs have been identified as high alert drugs by the Institute for Safe Medication Practices (ISMP's). Studies have confirmed that sedatives are among the highest- risk medications for adverse drug events. Sedatives because of a narrow therapeutic range or inherent toxic nature; have a high risk of causing devastating injury or death if improperly prescribed, dispensed, administered, monitored or stored. Therefore, special attention and extra care are needed when dealing with sedative drugs in critical care settings. Medication management processes including sedatives consist of three main stages: prescribing, dispensing, and administrating, although some researchers specified additional steps such as monitoring, storage and reporting [55, 90-97].

Sedative drugs prescription is normally the responsibility of the ICU physician and critical care nurses normally manage the dose and frequency. Critical care nurse's goal is to ensure that patients receive sedatives as they have been prescribed. Nurses seen as the main defense against prescribing errors, as they check the drug charts continuously [97-99].

Critical care nurses are responsible for determining that each medication order is complete with a legible drug name, dose with appropriate units of measurement, route and frequency. The appropriateness of a sedative for a patient should be assessed by taking into consideration the details of the current health problem; co-existing and past medical history such as respiratory and cardiovascular disorders; because many sedative drugs tend to cause significant cardiovascular and respiratory depression. History of allergies must be assessed, especially if the patient has hypersensitivity to previous sedation or anesthetic medications or if there is allergies to eggs or soy products for propofol (diprivan) [100-103].

Critical care nurses must check the results of relevant investigations such as serum triglyceride levels for propofol (diprivan) if used for more than 48 hrs, or hepatic and renal function for diazepam (neuril) during prolonged therapy. Current medications must be checked, especially if there are combination between sedatives and opioids, because the opioids have respiratory depressant and other adverse effects and may be potentially dangerous synergistic effects when they are used in combination with sedatives. The time and nature of last meal either liquid or solid must be checked for the patients undergoing procedural sedation to minimize the potential risk of aspiration [55, 66, 100-103].

Sedatives dispension includes the selection, preparation and transfer of a medication to patients for administration. In some settings, medication orders are transcribed, dispensed, and then delivered for nurse administration. In certain circumstances and settings, both nurses and pharmacists are involved in transcribing, dispensing, and delivering medications. Critical care nurses should compare medication, container label, and medication record. Double-checks have been reported to have significantly reduced the incident rate of dispensing errors. Propofol is available in both 1 and 2 per cent concentrations, so labels should be checked especially carefully. Critical care nurses should have a clear understanding of the different names used because the drugs may have several names assigned to them; a generic name and a trade name. This is confusing especially when the names sound similar or the spellings are similar; for examples critical care nurses shouldn't confuse versed with vepesid or diazepam with lorazepam [20, 56, 96, 99, 104, 105].

Critical care nurses should maintain aseptic technique during sedative drugs dispensing especially for propofol. This includes washing hands, wearing gloves, disinfecting the neck of the ampoule or the rubber stopper of the vial before use, using careful technique when preparing a syringe of the medication immediately before use, restricting the use of an ampoule or vial to a single patient and discarding all unused portions of medication and IV infusion set after 12 hrs if administered directly from vial or after 6 hrs if transferred to a syringe or other container. If propofol dilution is necessary, only dextrose-5%-water (D_5W) should be used, and should be shaken well before use and the bottle should be inspected visually for particulate matter and discoloration. All these precautions are essential during the handling of propofol to prevent extrinsic contamination and dangerous infectious complications. For midazolam, if dilution is necessary, D_5W or 0.9% NaCl can be used [55, 66, 105].

Sedatives administration is an integral part of nursing duties. Accurate administration of sedatives is critically dependent on the quality of all of the previous steps, which include the prescribing and dispensing processes. Critical care nurse should identify the patient and must be certain that the patient receiving the drug is the patient for whom the drug has been ordered. This is accomplished by checking the patient's wristband containing the patient's name. If there is no written identification verifying the patient's name, critical care nurses obtain a wristband or other form of identification before administering the drug [21, 55, 56, 93].

Sedation assessment can be 'buried' amongst the myriad of other assessment critical care nurses undertake in their daily care. Nursing assessment of sedation is an assessment that involves both consideration of patient behaviour, general appearance, response to verbal and physical stimuli, and more objective observations including respiratory rate, oxygen saturation, heart rate and rhythm, blood pressure and level of consciousness [21, 55].

Critical care nurses must determine the minimum level of sedation required, which should be clarified at the beginning of ICU care and reassessed on a regular basis as the patient's clinical condition changes. Use of sedation scale allows the physician to set an optimal level of sedation for their patients and provides critical care nurses with a goal for medication titration to achieve this level. In the absence of tools, assessing the adequacy of sedation can be problematic because of its largely subjective nature. It is a bedside procedure in which critical care nurses participation is vital. Critical care nurses frequently note changes in the patients' optimal level of sedation because they are present at the bedside continuously. Infusions of any paralysing agents should be stopped long enough before sedation assessment to ensure they will not influence results [4, 21, 83, 104, 106].

Sedation of agitated critically ill patients should be started only after providing adequate analgesia. Therefore, critical care nurses should assess the level of pain to rule out any sensation of pain. Pain should be monitored with a tool that permits the patient to indicate the level of pain regardless of their ability to vocalize. A visual analogue scale or numeric rating scale can be applied in the ICU and will assist significantly in assessing the level of pain control. Patients who cannot communicate should be assessed through subjective observation of pain-related behaviors such as movement, facial expression, posturing, and physiological indicators such as respiratory rate, heart rate and blood pressure [4].

Non pharmacological or environmental strategies must be considered by Critical care nurses to assist with management of sedated critically ill patients. Critical care nurses must be creative in developing that method including environmental control such as humidity, temperature, lighting and noise. Critical care nurses must also provide the patient and family members' with constant reassurance, repetitive feedback, frequent communication and explanation to assists in calming fears and anxiousness. Other interventions must be implemented by critical care nurses include massage, frequent repositioning, oral care, and diversion activities such as listening to music or having a family member nearby [4, 26, 30, 107].

Critical care nurses are legally responsible for applying and ensuring the "five rights" of drug administration, which include the right patient, the right drug, the right dosage, the right time, and the right route. Other institutions have adopted the right for monitoring, as well as documentation and patient education, as crucial, complementary steps to the "five rights check" [92, 94, 108].

However, nursing responsibilities do not rely only on these five rights when administering sedatives. Titrating sedatives presents a significant challenge to nursing staff at the patients' bedside. Titrating dosages of sedation is similar to prescribing medication in that it requires of critical care nurses comprehensive knowledge of the drug, its potential side effects and interactions with other medications, and its impact on an individual's physiological condition. Critical care nurses spend a considerable amount of time at their patient's bedside continuously assessing their need for sedation, evaluating their progress and intervening in a timely manner to maintain stability. Critical care nurses increase or decrease the rate of infusion within the prescribed range according to the level of sedation and the patient's need [21, 45].

When the intravenous route is used, securing venous access is mandatory, and specific antagonist drugs, if available, must be at hand. Intravenous access should be continuously maintained to administer sedation and to reverse any undesired effects. Some sedative drugs such as diazepam may cause phlebitis and venous thrombosis. Therefore, critical care nurses must assess the intravenous site frequently during sedatives administration [55].

Critical care nurses must dispose unusable portions of medications in an appropriate manner and returning drugs that require special storage to the storage area immediately after they are prepared for administration. This rule applies mainly to the refrigeration of drugs but may also apply to drugs that must be protected from exposure to light or heat. Diazepam (neuril) should not be stored in plastic syringe and continuous infusion is not recommended because addition of diazepam to an IV infusion solution or plastic syringes may result in adsorption of diazepam to the plastic container and tubing [20, 55, 105, 109].

Sedation monitoring is an important component of nursing care in the ICU. Critical care nurses in their role of monitoring patients are in a position to provide valuable input in the selection of the most desirable sedative drug. Critical care nurses should monitor patients during and after sedative administration for expected benefits and adverse effects, and intervene as necessary. The level of sedation, level of consciousness, oxygen saturation, heart rate and blood pressure should be monitored continuously by critical care nurses. Continuous monitoring and assessing patients' level of sedation is complex without a framework on which to base an assessment. Sedation scoring tools provide a framework for evaluating the effectiveness of sedation administered to individual patients. Despite that the vital signs are not sensitive markers of sedation but many of adverse outcomes associated with sedatives administration can be reduced with early detection of changes in oxygen saturation, heart rate and blood pressure that lead to interventions to avert serious problems. In addition, critical care nurses should institute fall prevention strategies such as maintaining bed side rails elevated [55, 110].

Documentation is a critical element of drug administration. Effective documentation promotes continuity of care; establishes accountability; enhances communication between critical care nurses and other healthcare providers. Appropriate documentation of sedative administered includes sedative name; date and time of administration; dose; route and/or site; allergy assessment and signature of the critical care nurse who has administered the sedative. Sedation scales can be used to define the goals of sedation as well as to help simplify documentation. Also, when titrating sedation the sedation scale and the corresponding infusion rate should be documented on the nursing flow sheet. Also, critical care nurses should notify the physician immediately for any adverse reactions, complications, or side effects such as respiratory depression, hypotension or changes in the patient's general medical condition prior to and/or after administration of the sedation medication [41, 99, 110 - 111].

Achieving and maintaining a specific sedation goal requires nursing vigilance. Patient response to medication is often unpredictable and varies not only within and between patient populations, but also within a single hospital stay for an individual patient. Drug accumulation, changes in hemodynamic status, changes in renal, endocrine, and liver function, and the effects of drug to drug interaction can increase or decrease the effectiveness of sedative agents. Therefore, a firm understanding of the clinical pharmacology of these agents is imperative for their optimal use in critical care setting [28, 112, 113].

Aim of the study

The aim of this study is to identify critical care nurses' knowledge and practices regarding the safe use of sedatives.

Research question

What are the critical care nurses' knowledge and practices regarding the safe use of sedatives?

Chapter III

Materials&Method

Materials and Method

Materials

Research design

A descriptive design was used in this study.

Settings

This study was conducted in the casualty intensive care unit (Unit I) which contains fifteen beds and the general intensive care unit (Unit III) which contains sixteen beds, at the Alexandria Main University Hospital.

Subjects

A convenient sample of fifty critical care nurses including technical, and intern nurses who were involved in providing direct patient care throughout the three different shifts (morning, evening and night) in the previously mentioned units were included in this study.

Tools

Two tools were used for data collection.

Tool one: "Safe Use of Sedatives Observation Checklist"(appendix II)

This tool was developed by the researcher after reviewing the related literature [4, 55, 90, 96, 110, 114-117] to assess critical care nurses' practices regarding sedative drugs administration. It consists of three parts:

Part I: "Demographic data"

It includes the name of the ICU, the shifts (morning, evening and night), and patient's sex and age.

Part II: "Clinical data"

It includes clinical data in relation to sedation including admission medical diagnosis, presence of attached machines, indication(s) for sedatives, sedative drugs used and routes of administration.

Part III: "Sedative use practices"

It includes five sections as follows:

1. **Prescription** which includes sedative's name, dose, unit, route, method of administration, frequency and infusion type. It includes also checking the patient's chart for current medications, medical history, allergies, time and nature of last oral intake and laboratory investigations.

2. **Dispensing** which includes washing hands, maintaining aseptic technique, checking the expiration date, comparing sedative with physician's order, avoiding mixing sedative with other drugs and considering special nursing precautions for each sedative drug.

3. **Administering** which includes identifying the patient, setting target level of sedation in collaboration with physician, assessing the IV site for inflammation/irritation. It includes also administering of the sedative according the route of administration such as administering continuous intravenous infusion by syringe pump, drip infusion or IV bolus injection, ensuring patency of IV line, titrating sedative according to sedation scale and discarding disposable equipment. In addition to considering non-pharmacological strategies such as explaining the procedure, communicating clearly, providing verbal assurance, adjusting the light and controlling the noise.

4. **Monitoring** which includes level of sedation, level of pain, level of consciousness, respiratory rate, oxygen saturation, heart rate, heart rhythm and blood pressure.

5. **Documentation and reporting** which includes documentation of pre-procedural assessment, sedative's name, dose, route, method of administration, time, date, flow rate, monitoring parameters and adverse sedative reactions. It includes also reporting of adverse sedative reactions especially respiratory complications such as hypoxia and aspiration, cardiovascular complications such as dysrhythmia or for other adverse sedative reactions and if target sedation level is not achieved.

Each item in this part is scored as follows:

- The task which is performed completely/accurately is graded as two points.

- The task which is performed incorrect/incomplete is graded as one point.

- The task which is not done is graded as zero.

The cut point for "Good" is ≥75% of the total score, "Fair" is between 50% to less than 75% of the total score, and "Poor" is less than 50% of the total score.

Tool two: "Safe Use of Sedatives Structured Questionnaire" (appendix II)

This tool was developed by the researcher after reviewing the related literature [4, 34, 55, 68] to assess critical care nurses' knowledge in relation to safe use of sedatives. It consists of three parts:

Part I: "Critical care nurses' characteristics"

It includes demographic data of critical care nurses including: sex, age, level of education, job title, years of experience and source(s) of information regarding sedative drugs.

Part II: "Self report of current sedation practices"

It includes four questions about critical care nurses self report of current sedation practices, such as use of sedation protocol or guidelines, methods of sedation level determination and methods of continuous IV sedation discontinuation.

Part III: "Critical care nurses' knowledge regarding safe use of sedatives"

This part covers 61 questions distributed into nine main categories to assess critical care nurses' knowledge regarding safe use of sedatives. Two types of questions were used; multiple choice questions and true/false questions. The total number of multiple choice questions was nineteen and the total number of true/false questions was forty two, these nine categories were as follows:

- **Sedative drugs names**; which includes three true/false questions.
- **Sedative drugs action and pharmacokinetics**; which includes eight questions, four of them are multiple choice questions and four true/false questions.
- **Indications of sedatives**; which includes eight true/false questions.
- **Side effects of sedative drugs**; which includes five questions, one multiple choice question and four true/false questions.
- **Complications of sedation**; which includes six true/false questions.
- **General precautions of sedative drugs**; which include five questions, two of them are multiple choice questions and three true/false questions.
- **Special precautions of sedative drugs**; which includes thirteen questions; seven of them multiple choice questions and six true/false questions.
- **Sedation monitoring**; which includes ten questions; four of them are multiple choice questions and six true/false questions.
- **Documentation and reporting**: which includes three questions; one of them is multiple choice question and two true/false questions.

- The answer of each knowledge question is scored as follows:

    - The correct response scored as "1" and incorrect response scored as "0".
    - The cut point for "Good" is ≥75% of the total score, "Fair" is between 50% to less than 75% of the total score, and "Poor" is less than 50% of the total score.

Method

1. An official letter was directed from the Faculty of Nursing in Alexandria University to hospital administrative authority in order to obtain their acceptance to collect the necessary data from the selected ICUs. Then, the permission was obtained from the hospital administrative authority after providing an explanation of the study aim.

2. Safe use of sedatives observation checklist (Tool I) and safe use of sedatives structured questionnaire (Tool II) were developed by the researcher after reviewing the related literature [4, 34, 55, 68 90, 96, 110, 114-117].

3. Safe use of sedatives structured questionnaire (Tool II) was developed in Arabic by the researcher based on reviewing the related literature.

4. Both tools of the study were tested for content validity by seven experts in the fields of critical care nursing and pharmacy. Three of them were professors and one of them was assistant professor of critical care nursing in the Faculty of Nursing. In addition to three professors of pharmacy in the Faculty of Pharmacy at Alexandria University. Accordingly, all necessary modifications were done.

5. Ethical issues:

   - The researcher explained to the critical care nurses the objectives of the study orally, additionally to the written explanations on the covering letter of the questionnaire.

   - The anonymity and confidentiality of responses, voluntary participation and right to refuse to participate in the study was emphasized to critical care nurses.

6. A pilot study was conducted on ten critical care nurses to test the clarity, applicability and feasibility of the developed tools; they were excluded from the total sample. Accordingly, all necessary modifications were done.

7. Safe use of sedatives structured questionnaire (Tool II) was tested for its reliability by using Cronbach's coefficient alpha, the reliability coefficients were ($r = 0.72$) which is acceptable.

8. Data collection:

   - Safe use of sedatives observation checklist (Tool I) was used to observe critical care nurse's practices regarding the safe use of sedatives. Each nurse involved in providing direct patients care was observed individually by the researcher for safe use of sedatives three times over the different three shifts (morning, evening and night) once during each shift.

- After finishing all observations; safe use of sedatives structured questionnaire (Tool II) was distributed to the critical care nurses who were observed to assess critical care nurses' knowledge in relation to safe use of sedatives. Critical care nurses were asked to answer the questionnaire and to bring it back to the researcher at the end of the shift. The researcher was available to clarify any question.

- Data were collected by the researcher during approximately three months starting from 10th of January 2012 to 5th of April 2012).

Statistical analysis

The raw data were coded and transformed into coding sheets. The results were checked. Then, the data were entered into SPSS system files (SPSS package version 18) using personal computer. Output drafts were checked against the revised coded data for typing and spelling mistakes. Finally, analysis and interpretation of data were conducted.

The following statistical measures were used:

- Descriptive statistics including frequency, distribution, mean, and standard deviation were used to describe different characteristics.
- Kolmogorov – Smirnov test was used to examine the normality of data distribution.
- Univariate analyses including: t-test, and ANOVA test were used to test the significance of results of quantitative variables.
- Chi-square test and Monte Carlo test were used to test the significance of results of qualitative variables.
- Pearson correlation was conducted to show relation between knowledge and practice scores.
- The significance of the results was at the 5% level of significance.

Limitations of study

This study was conducted in two ICUs and therefore the results cannot be generalized as the sample is convenient, sample size, not geography distribution and not represent all population.

Chapter IV

Results

RESULTS

The aim of this study is to identify critical care nurses' knowledge and practices regarding the safe use of sedatives. The results are divided into six parts as follows:

> ***Part 1:*** Critical care nurses' characteristics (***table 1, figure 6***)
>
> ***Part 2:*** Critical care nurses' self report of current sedation practices (***table 2***)

Part 1: Critical care nurses' characteristics

Table (1) shows the distribution of critical care nurses according to their characteristics. In relation to **demographic data**, more than half of critical care nurses (58%) are females and the majority of them (88%) are between 20 to less than 25 years old. More than three quarters of critical care nurses (76.0%) hold a bachelor degree of nursing, and the rest of them (24.0%) hold a diploma degree.

In relation to **job-related data**, it shows that more than half of critical care nurses (54.0%) are working in casualty care unit (unit I), while the rest of them are working in general care unit (unit III). In relation to job title, it was found that most of the nurses (76.0%) are intern nurses, and the rest of them (24.0%) are technical nurses. Regarding critical care nurses' years of experience in critical care units in the hospital, about two thirds of the critical care nurses (64.0 %) have an experience of less than one year, and for 18.0% of them, it ranges between 1 to less than 5 years, and the remaining 18.0% have an experience ranges between 5 to less than 10 years.

Table (1): Distribution of critical care nurses according to their characteristics

Critical care nurses' characteristics	Nurses (n=50)	
	No.	**%**
Demographic data		
Sex		
• Male	21	42.0
• Female	29	58.0
Age (years)		
• 20 < 25	44	88.0
• 25 < 30	6	12.0
Educational level		
• Bachelor degree	38	76.0
• Diploma degree	12	24.0
Job-related data		
ICU		
• Casualty ICU (unit I)	27	54.0
• General ICU (unit III)	23	46.0
Job title		
• Nurse supervisor (intern)	38	76.0
• Technical nurse	12	24.0
Experience in ICU (years)		
• Less than 1	32	64.0

• 1< 5	9	18.0
• 5 < 10	9	18.0

Figure (6) reflects the distribution of the critical care nurses according to source(s) of information regarding sedatives. It demonstrates that, the majority of critical care nurses (88.0%) had information from the practical experience, and more than half of them (56.0%) had information from undergraduate courses. Slightly less than one third of critical care nurses (30.0%) had information from search in the internet, while only 4.0% of them had information from scientific conferences and workshops.

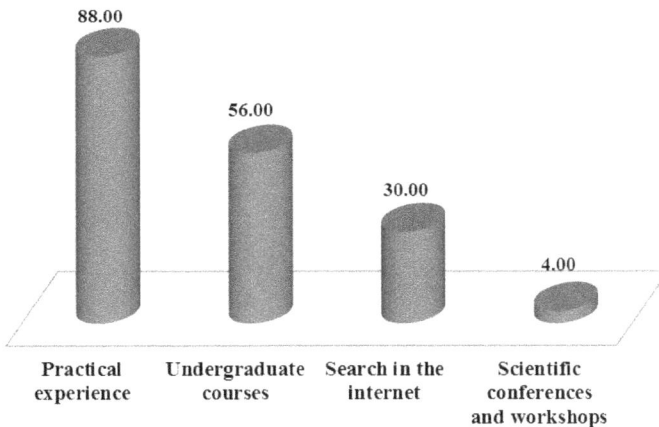

#Categories are not mutually exclusive

Figure (6): Distribution of critical care nurses according to source(s) of information regarding sedatives

Part 2: Critical care nurses' self report of current sedation practices

Table (2) illustrates the distribution of critical care nurses according to self report of current sedation practices. In relation to use of **sedation protocol/guidelines**, all critical care nurses (100.0%) reported that they did not use any sedation protocol. Concerning the **methods of sedation level determination**, all critical care nurses (100.0%) reported that they

41

did not use any *subjective sedation scale* to determine the level of sedation and nearly half of critical care nurses (44.0%) reported that they use the *vital signs* as an *objective method* to determine level of sedation, while the rest of them (56.0%) did not use vital signs to determine level of sedation.

In relation to **methods of continuous sedatives IV infusion discontinuation**, it is clear that all critical care nurses (100.0%) reported use of gradual method, and in relation to this method; about one third of critical care nurses (32.0%) reported use of gradual sedatives withdrawal over several days, and slightly more than one third of them (34.0%) reported use of gradual sedatives withdrawal throughout the day, while only 12.0 of critical care nurses reported use of gradual sedatives withdrawal throughout the shift.

Table (2): Distribution of critical care nurses according to self report of current sedation practices

Self report of current sedation practices	Nurses (n=50)	
	No.	%
Use of sedation protocol/ guidelines		
• Used	0	0.0
• Not used	50	100.0
Methods of sedation level determination		
− **Subjective method**		
• Sedation scale		
− Used	0	0.0
− Not used	50	100.0
− **Objective method**		
• Vital signs		
− Used	22	44.0
− Not used	28	56.0
Methods of continuous IV sedation discontinuation		
• Gradual	50	100.0
• Abrupt	0	0.0

Methods of gradual sedatives withdrawal		
• Over several days (daily interruption)	16	32.0
• Throughout the day	17	34.0
• Throughout the shift	6	12.0
• Do not know	11	22.0

Part 3: Critical care nurses' knowledge regarding safe use of sedatives

Table (3) shows distribution of critical care nurses' knowledge regarding sedatives names, action and pharmacokinetics. **Concerning generic name**, the majority of critical care nurses (86.0%) knew the generic name of propofol, and more than half of them (54.0%) knew the generic name of midazolam, while about two thirds of critical care nurses (66.0%) did not know the generic name of diazepam.

Regarding sedatives **action and pharmacokinetics**, in relation to propofol, about two thirds of critical care nurses (66.0%) did not know that *propofol* have anxiolytic effects, while slightly less than three quarters of them (74.0%) knew that the patient wakes up quickly after discontinuation of propofol. Concerning *midazolam*, slightly less than two thirds of critical care nurses (64.0%) knew that midazolam have amnestic properties, and more than half of them (58.0%) did not know that midazolam have anxiolytic effects. Regarding *diazepam*, half of critical care nurses (50.0%) knew that diazepam does not have analgesic properties. Only 36.0% of critical care nurses knew that *diazepam, midazolam and propofol* did not have analgesic properties.

Table (3): Distribution of critical care nurses' knowledge regarding sedatives' names, action and pharmacokinetics

Sedative names action and pharmacokinetics	Nurses' knowledge (n=50)			
	Know		Do not know	
	No.	%	No.	%
Generic name				
• Propofol	43	86.0	7	14.0
• Midazolam	27	54.0	23	46.0
• Diazepam	17	34.0	33	66.0
Mean± S.D= 58±26.2				
Action and pharmacokinetics				
Propofol (*diprivan*):				
• Have anxiolytic effects	17	34.0	33	66.0
• Patient is wakes up quickly	37	74.0	13	26.0

Sedative names action and pharmacokinetics	Nurses' knowledge (n=50)			
	Know		Do not know	
	No.	%	No.	%
• Preferred for weaning	25	50.0	25	50.0
Midazolam (*dormicum*): • Have amnestic properties	32	<u>64.0</u>	18	36.0
• Have anxiolytic effects	21	42.0	29	<u>58.0</u>
• Peak effect between 2-5 minutes	26	52.0	24	48.0
Diazepam (*neuril, valium*): • Does not have analgesic properties	25	<u>50.0</u>	25	50.0
Diazepam, midazolam and propofol do not have analgesic properties	18	<u>36.0</u>	32	64.0
Mean± S.D = 50.3±17.0				

Table (4) shows distribution of critical care nurses' knowledge regarding indications of sedatives. In relation to **injury prevention**, more than three quarters of critical care nurses (76.0%) knew that sedatives are indicated to reduce patients' anxiety, agitation and delirium. Regarding **medical goals facilitation,** more than two thirds of critical care nurses (68.0%) did not know that sedatives are indicated to promote sleep and three fifths of them (60.0%) did not know that sedatives are indicated to maintain patient/ventilator synchrony. While more than half of critical care nurses knew that sedatives are indicated to decrease intracranial pressure and to decrease oxygen consumption (54.0%, 54.0% respectively). Concerning **humanitarian intentions**, more than two thirds of critical care nurses (70.0%) did not know that sedatives are indicated to induce amnesia, while more than two thirds of critical care nurses (70.0%) knew that sedatives are indicated to decrease stress related to procedures.

Table (4): Distribution of critical care nurses' knowledge regarding indications of sedatives

Indications of sedatives	Nurses' knowledge (n=50)			
	Know		Do not know	
	No.	%	No.	%
Injury prevention: • Reduce anxiety, agitation and delirium	38	<u>76.0</u>	12	24.0
• Prevent patients' risk of self harm	29	58.0	21	42.0
Medical goals facilitation: • Promote sleep	16	32.0	34	<u>68.0</u>
• Maintain patient /ventilator synchrony	20	40.0	30	<u>60.0</u>
• Decrease oxygen consumption	27	<u>54.0</u>	23	46.0
• Decrease intracranial pressure	27	<u>54.0</u>	23	46.0

Indications of sedatives	Nurses' knowledge (n=50)			
	Know		Do not know	
	No.	%	No.	%
Humanitarian intentions: • Induce amnesia	15	30.0	35	<u>70.0</u>
• Decrease stress related to procedures	35	<u>70.0</u>	15	30.0
Mean± S.D = 51.8±19.7				

Table (5) reflects distribution of critical care nurses' knowledge regarding side effects of sedatives. In relation to **propofol**, more than half of critical care nurses (54.0%) knew that the most common side effect of propofol is hypotension. Regarding **midazolam,** three fifths of critical care nurses knew that side effects of midazolam include hypotension, respiratory depression, apnea and delirium (60.0%, 60.0% respectively), while slightly more than three fifths of them (62.0%) did not know that midazolam may cause paradoxical reactions such as agitation and restlessness in some patients. Concerning **diazepam**, half of critical care nurses (50.0%) knew that diazepam may cause local irritation at IV site.

Table (5): Distribution of critical care nurses' knowledge regarding side effects of sedatives

Side effects of sedatives	Nurses' knowledge (n=50)			
	Know		Do not know	
	No.	%	No.	%
Propofol (_diprivan_) : • Hypotension	27	<u>54.0</u>	23	46.0
Midazolam (_dormicum_): • Hypotension, respiratory depression and apnea	30	<u>60.0</u>	20	40.0
• Delirium	30	<u>60.0</u>	20	40.0
• Paradoxical reactions (agitation and restlessness)	19	38.0	31	<u>62.0</u>
Diazepam (_neuril, valium_) : • Local irritation at IV site	25	<u>50.0</u>	25	50.0
Mean± S.D = 48.4±23.9				

Table (6) shows distribution of critical care nurses' knowledge regarding complications of sedation. In relation to **complications related to level of sedation**, More than three quarters of critical care nurses (76.0%) knew that oversedation hinders accurate nervous system assessment, while slightly less than two thirds of them (64.0%) did not know that oversedation prolongs the duration of mechanical ventilation. Three fifths of critical care nurses (60%) knew that undersedation increase the heart rate and blood pressure

Regarding **complications related to methods of administration,** about two thirds of critical care nurses (66.0%) knew that administration of sedatives by continuous IV infusion prolongs duration of mechanical ventilation, and more than half of them (58.0%) knew that continuous IV sedatives infusion hinders accurate assessment of level of consciousness (LOC). Three fifths of critical care nurses (60.0%) knew that abrupt discontinuation of IV infusion cause withdrawal symptoms such as hypertension, and agitation.

Table (6): Distribution of critical care nurses' knowledge regarding complications of sedation

Complications of sedation	Nurses' knowledge (n=50)			
	Know		Do not know	
	No.	%	No.	%
Complications related to level of sedation - Oversedation: • *Hinder nervous system assessment*	38	<u>76.0</u>	12	24.0
• *Prolong mechanical ventilation*	18	36.0	32	<u>64.0</u>
- Undersedation • *Increased heart rate & blood pressure*	30	<u>60.0</u>	20	40.0
Complications related to methods of administration - Continuous IV infusion • *Prolong mechanical ventilation*	33	<u>66.0</u>	17	34.0
• *Hinder accurate assessment of LOC*	29	<u>58.0</u>	21	42.0
- Abrupt discontinuation of IV infusion • *Cause withdrawal symptoms (hypertension, agitation)*	30	<u>60.0</u>	20	40.0
Mean± S.D = 59.4±12.0				

Table (7) presents distribution of critical care nurses' knowledge regarding sedative precautions. In relation to sedative **general precautions**, more than half of critical care nurses (56.0%) knew that the informed consent should be obtained for procedural sedation, and slightly more than three fifths of critical care nurses (62.0%) knew that the level of pain should be determined in sedated critically ill patients. More than half of critical care nurses (56.0%) knew that the neuromuscular blocking agents must be discontinued prior to assessment of the level of sedation, while more than two thirds of them (70.0%) did not know that daily interruption of sedatives should be implemented during sedatives discontinuation.

In relation to sedative **special precautions**, concerning *prescription*, more than half of critical care nurses (52.0%) knew that propofol is contraindicated if there are allergies to eggs or soybeans, while the majority of them (82.0%) did not know that diazepam is contraindicated to patients with shock and coma. Regarding *dispensing*, more than three quarters of critical care nurses (78.0%) did not know that propofol requires a dedicated IV infusion set and more than two thirds of them (68.0%) did not know that IV infusion set must be changed every 12 hrs. Slightly less than three quarters of critical care nurses (74.0%) knew that the midazolam should be diluted with D5W or 0.9% NaCl, while the vast majority of them (92.0%) did not know that diazepam should not be stored in a plastic syringe.

Concerning *administration*, slightly less than three fifths of critical care nurses (58.0%) did not know that propofol should be administered within 12 hrs. Less than two thirds of critical care nurses knew that the calories should be calculated during propofol administration and knew that diazepam should be administered slowly by IV bolus injection (64.0%, 64.0% respectively). Slightly less than three fifths of critical care nurses (58.0%) did not know that diazepam antagonist is flumazenil and more than half of them (56.0%) did not know that midazolam antagonist is flumazenil.

Table (7): Distribution of critical care nurses' knowledge regarding sedative precautions

Sedative precautions	Nurses' knowledge (n=50)			
	Know		Do not know	
	No.	%	No.	%
General precautions				
• Obtaining informed consent for procedural sedation	28	56.0	22	44.0
• Fasting for 8 hrs before elective procedure	25	50.0	25	50.0
• etermining pain level	31	62.0	19	38.0
• Discontinuing neuromuscular blocking agents	28	56.0	22	44.0
• Daily interruption of sedatives infusion	15	30.0	35	70.0
Mean± S.D = 50.8±12.3				
Special precautions				

Sedative precautions	Nurses' knowledge (n=50)			
	Know		Do not know	
	No.	%	No.	%
Prescription:				
• _Propofol_ is contraindicated if there are allergies to eggs/ soybeans	26	52.0	24	48.0
• _Diazepam_ is contraindicated to patients with shock/coma	9	18.0	41	82.0
Dispensing:				
• _Propofol_ • Should be diluted with D5W	20	40.0	30	60.0
• IV infusion set must be changed every 12 hrs	16	32.0	34	68.0
• Require dedicated IV infusion set	11	22.0	39	78.0
• Require aseptic techniques during handling	20	40.0	30	60.0
• _Midazolam_ should be diluted with D5W or 0.9% NaCl	37	74.0	13	26.0
• _Diazepam_ not recommended to storing in a plastic syringe	4	8.0	46	92.0
Administration:				
• _Propofol_ • Should be administered within 12 hrs	21	42.0	29	58.0
• Calories should be calculated during administration	32	64.0	18	36.0
• _Diazepam_ • Should be administered slowly for IV injection	32	64.0	18	36.0
• Antagonist is flumazenil	21	42.0	29	58.0
• _Midazolam_ antagonist is flumazenil	22	44.0	28	56.0
Mean± S.D = 41.7±14.3				

Table (8) reveals distribution of critical care nurses' knowledge regarding sedation monitoring. Regarding **monitoring parameters**, more than two thirds of critical care nurses (68.0%) knew that the level of pain should be monitored, while more than three quarters of them (76.0%) did not know that QT interval should be monitored during haloperidol administration. Slightly more than two thirds of critical care nurses (70.0%) did not know that decrease in respiratory rate and hypoxia may indicate that the patient is oversedated, while more than half of them (56.0%) knew that unresponsiveness may indicate oversedation, and three fifths of critical care nurses knew that the increase of heart rate and blood pressure may indicate that the patient is undersedated (60.0%, 60.0% respectively). More than two thirds of critical care nurses (70.0%) knew signs and symptoms of sedatives withdrawal such as hypertension and agitation.

In relation to **duration of monitoring,** slightly less than two thirds of critical care nurses (64.0%) did not know the minimum monitoring time required after administration of sedatives antagonist, while more than half of them (54.0%) knew that monitoring time increased after procedural sedation.

Table (8): Distribution of critical care nurses' knowledge regarding sedation monitoring

Sedation monitoring	Nurses' knowledge (n=50)			
	Know		Do not know	
	No.	%	No.	%
Monitoring parameters: • Pain level	34	68.0	16	32.0
• Triglyceride level (for propofol > 48 hrs)	20	40.0	30	60.0
• ECG rhythm (QT interval for haloperidol)	12	24.0	38	76.0
• Signs of oversedation : – *Decrease respiratory rate and hypoxia*	15	30.0	35	70.0
– *Unresponsiveness*	28	56.0	22	44.0
• Signs of undersedation : – *Increase in heart rate*	30	60.0	20	40.0
– *Increase in blood pressure*	30	60.0	20	40.0
• Withdrawal symptoms: – *Hypertension, agitation and sleep disorder*	35	70.0	15	30.0
Monitoring duration: • Monitor patient for at least 2 hrs after administration of sedatives antagonist	18	36.0	32	64.0
• Increase monitoring time after procedural sedation	27	54.0	23	46.0
Mean± S.D = 49.8±15.3				

Table (9) shows distribution of critical care nurses' knowledge regarding documentation and reporting. More than half of critical care nurses (58.0%) did not know that monitoring parameters should be documented every 15 minutes after procedural sedation. The majority of critical care nurses (86.0%) knew that reporting to physicians should be done in case of hypoxia and more than two thirds of them (68.0%) knew that reporting to physicians should be done in case of aspiration.

Table (9): Distribution of critical care nurses' knowledge regarding documentation and reporting

Documentation and reporting	Nurses' knowledge (n=50)			
	Know		Do not know	
	No.	%	No.	%
Document: • Monitoring parameters every 15 minutes after	21	42.0	29	58.0

Documentation and reporting	Nurses' knowledge (n=50)			
	Know		Do not know	
	No.	%	No.	%
procedural sedation				
Report : • Hypoxia	43	<u>86.0</u>	7	14.0
• Aspiration	34	<u>68.0</u>	16	32.0
Mean± S.D = 65.3±24.3				

Table (10) indicates distribution of critical care nurses' mean percentage of knowledge regarding safe use of sedatives. It was found that critical care nurses had a fair level of knowledge in relation to sedative names, action, indications, complications, general precautions and documentations and reporting, while critical care nurses had a poor level of knowledge in relation to side effects of sedatives, special precautions and sedation monitoring.

Table (10): Distribution of critical care nurses' mean percentage of knowledge regarding safe use of sedatives

Knowledge	Mean ±SD
Sedative names	58.0±26.2
Sedatives action and pharmacokinetics	50.3±17.0
Side effects of sedatives	48.4±23.9
Indications of sedatives	51.8±19.7
Complications of sedation	59.4±12.0
General precautions of sedatives	50.8±12.3
Special precautions of sedatives	41.7±14.3
Sedation monitoring	49.8±15.3
Documentations and reporting	65.3±24.3
Total score	50.6±6.7

Part 4: Clinical data regarding sedation practices' in ICU

Figure (7) shows the distribution of sedated critically ill patients according to admission medical diagnosis. It reveals that 26.0% of patients had respiratory disorders, and 15.3% of them had cardiac disorders and neurological disorders respectively.

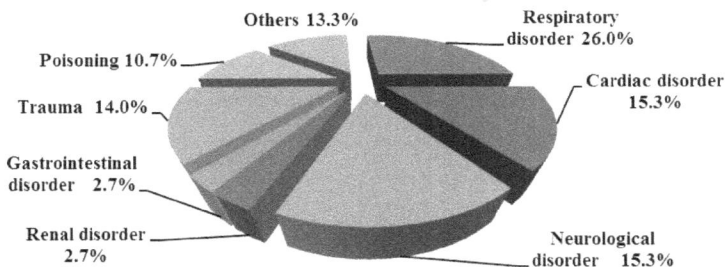

Figure (7): Distribution of sedated critically ill patients according to admission medical diagnosis

Table (11) shows the distribution of sedated critically ill patients according to presence of attached machines. It reveals that the majority of the sedated critically ill patients (86.0%) were attached to mechanical ventilator, and the vast majority of them (98.7%) were attached to cardiac monitor. Slightly more than half of patients attached to cardiac monitor (50.7%) were monitored by pulse oximeter, and slightly more than two thirds of them (68.9%) were monitored by blood pressure cuff.

Table (11): Distribution of sedated critically ill patients according to presence of attached machines

Attached machines	Sedated critically ill patients (n=150)			
	Yes		No	
	No.	%	No.	%
Mechanical ventilator	129	86.0	21	14.0
Cardiac monitor	148	98.7	2	1.3
Pulse oximeter (n=148)	75	50.7	73	49.3
Blood pressure cuff (n=148)	102	68.9	46	31.1

#Categories are not mutually exclusive

51

Table (12) reflects the distribution of sedated critically ill patients according to indications of sedatives. In relation to **injury prevention**, the majority of patients (82.7%) were sedated to decrease their anxiety and agitation, and slightly more than two thirds of them (69.3%) were sedated to facilitate tolerance of endotracheal tube. Regarding **medical goals facilitation,** more than half of patients (53.3%) were sedated to decrease oxygen consumption, while only about one fifth of them (18.7%) were sedated to decrease intracranial pressure. Concerning **humanitarian intentions**, about one fifth of patients (19.3%) were sedated to induce amnesia, and less than two thirds of patients (22.7%) were sedated to decrease stress related to procedures.

Table (12): Distribution of sedated critically ill patients according to indications of sedatives

Indications of sedatives	Sedated critically ill patients (n=150)			
	Indicated		Not indicated	
	No.	%	No.	%
#*Injury prevention*:				
• educe anxiety and agitation	124	82.7	26	17.3
• Facilitate tolerance of endotracheal tube	104	69.3	46	30.7
# *Medical goals facilitation*:				
• Promote sleep	9	6.0	141	94.0
• Decrease oxygen consumption	80	53.3	70	46.7
• Decrease intracranial pressure	28	18.7	122	81.3
• Treat convulsions	12	8.0	138	92.0
# *Humanitarian intentions*:				
• Induce amnesia	29	19.3	121	80.7
• #Decrease stress related to procedures	34	22.7	116	77.3
− Endotracheal intubation	21	61.8	13	38.2
− Tracheostomy tube insertion	11	32.4	23	67.6
− Chest tube insertion	1	2.9	33	97.1
− Cardioversion	1	2.9	33	97.1

#Categories are not mutually exclusive

Table (13) reveals the distribution of sedated critically ill patients according to sedatives and methods of IV administration. *In relation to sedatives*, propofol was used in about two thirds of patients (63.3%); midazolam was used in about one quarter of patients (24.0%), while diazepam was used in only 12.7% of them. *Regarding the methods of IV administration*, the results show that slightly more than three fifths of sedatives (61.3%) were administered by continuous IV infusion, while the rest of them (38.7%) were administered by intermittent bolus IV injection. For methods of administration of each sedative, it can be seen that 57.9% of *propofol* was administered by continuous IV drip infusion, 86.1% of *midazolam* was administered by intermittent bolus IV injection, and *diazepam* was administered only by intermittent bolus IV injection.

Table (13): Distribution of sedated critically ill patients according to sedatives and methods of IV administration

Sedatives	Methods of IV administration						Total (n=150)	
	Continuous IV infusion (n=92)				Intermittent bolus IV injection (n=58)			
	Syringe pump		Drip infusion					
	No.	%	No.	%	No.	%	No.	%
Propofol	32	33.7	55	57.9	8	8.4	95	63.3
Midazolam	4	11.1	1	2.8	31	86.1	36	24.0
Diazepam	0	00.0	0	00.0	19	100.0	19	12.7
Total	36	24.0	56	37.3	58	38.7	150	100.0
(n=150)	61.3%				38.7%		100.0%	

Figure (8) shows the distribution of sedated critically ill patients according to their level of sedation. It reveals that about half of sedated critically ill patients (48.5%) were adequately sedated, while 29.5% of them were under sedated and the rest of them 22.0% were over sedated.

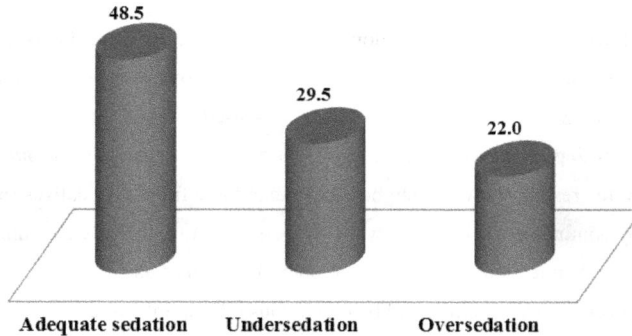

48.5   29.5   22.0

Adequate sedation   Undersedation   Oversedation

According to Ramsay sedation scale [29]: Score 1= undersedation   Score 2, 3, 4 or 5= adequate sedation

Score 6= over sedation

Figure (8): Distribution of sedated critically ill patients according to their level of sedation

Part 5: Critical care nurses' practices regarding safe use of sedatives

Table (14) shows the distribution of critical care nurses' practices regarding sedatives prescription. It can be noted that the majority of critical care nurses checked the physician order correctly throughout the three shifts (72.1%, 75.0%, and 80.5% respectively). More than half of critical care nurses did not check the current medications throughout the three shifts (61.1%, 56.3%, and 53.3% respectively). More than two thirds of critical care nurses did not check the patient's medical history throughout the three shifts (70.3%, 71.4% and 74.3% respectively). More than half of critical care nurses did not check the patient's history of allergy throughout the three shifts (51.6%, 56.3%, and 56.3% respectively).

All critical care nurses (100.0%) checked the time and nature of last meal for patients undergoing elective procedural sedation throughout the morning and night shifts, and three quarters of them (75.0%) checked it in the evening shift. None of the critical care nurses check the levels of triglyceride for propofol infusion throughout the three shifts. More than two thirds of critical care nurses did not administer analgesic drugs as physician's order or as needed in the evening and night shifts (70.0%, 65.5%, respectively), while half of them (50.0%) administered it in the morning shift.

From this table, it can be noted that there is a statistically significant differences between the three shifts only in checking the physician order (X^2=8.18, P=0.017), while there are no statistically significant differences between the three shifts in the other items.

Table (14): Distribution of critical care nurses' practices regarding sedatives prescription

Prescription	Morning						Evening						Night						Test of significance
	C/C		Inc/Inc		ND		C/C		Inc/Inc		ND		C/C		Inc/Inc		ND		
	No.	%	No.	%	No.	%	No.	%	No.	%	No.	%	No.	%	No.	%	No.	%	
Check: - Physician's order (drug's name, dose, unit, route, frequency and infusion type).	31	72.1	12	27.9	0	0.0	33	75.0	11	25.0	0	0.0	33	80.5	8	19.5	0	0.0	X^2=8.18 P=0.017*
- Current medications (opioids)	1	5.6	6	33.3	11	61.1	2	12.5	5	31.3	9	56.3	1	6.7	6	40.0	8	53.3	MCp=0.934
- Medical history	7	18.9	4	10.8	26	70.3	8	22.9	2	5.7	25	71.4	7	20.0	2	5.7	26	74.3	MCp=0.906
- Allergies	12	38.7	3	9.7	16	51.6	13	40.6	1	3.1	18	56.3	13	40.6	1	3.1	18	56.3	MCp=0.772
- Time/nature of last meal for elective procedure	4	100.0	0	0.0	0	0.0	3	75.0	0	0.0	1	25.0	4	100.0	0	0.0	0	0.0	MCp=0.457
Triglyceride level (if propofol used > 48 hrs)	0	0.0	0	0.0	23	100.0	0	0.0	0	0.0	27	100.0	0	0.0	0	0.0	26	100.0	-NA-
Administer analgesic drugs as physician's order / as needed	11	50.0	0	0.0	11	50.0	9	30.0	0	0.0	21	70.0	10	34.5	0	0.0	19	65.5	X^2=2.30 P=0.316
	Mean± S.D = 22.4±17.1						Mean± S.D = 21.6±14.9						Mean± S.D = 20.7±15.6						
							Mean± S.D (Average) = 21.6±12.0												

C / C: Correct or Complete   Inc / Inc: Incorrect or Incomplete   ND: Not done   NA: Not Applicable
X^2: Chi-square test   MCp: Monte Carlo test   *: Statistically significant at p ≤ 0.05
(If number and percentage in any item is less than what is expected, this means that it is not applicable)

55

Table (15 - a) reveals the distribution of critical care nurses' practices regarding sedatives dispensing. It can be noted that about two thirds of critical care nurses did not wash or disinfect their hands throughout the three shifts (62.0%, 64.0%, and 66.0% respectively). More than half of critical care nurses did not wear clean gloves during the handling of sedatives throughout the three shifts (54.0%, 58.0%, and 56.0% respectively). All critical care nurses (100.0%) checked correctly the prescribed sedatives (the first check) throughout the three shifts, and the majority of them perform the second check throughout the three shifts (84.0%, 82.0%, and 82.0% respectively). More than two thirds of critical care nurses did not compare the sedative with the physician's order in the morning and evening shifts (69.8%, 70.5%, respectively), and less than two thirds of them (63.4%) did not follow this step in the night shift. All critical care nurses (100.0%) avoided mixing sedatives with other medications. The vast majority of critical care nurses did not maintain aseptic technique during handling of sedatives throughout the three shifts (92.0%, 96.0%, and 90.0% respectively).

Table (15 - b) shows the distribution of critical care nurses' practices regarding **specific sedatives dispensing**. In relation to ***propofol***, it can be noted that the majority of critical care nurses did not inspect the bottle for particular matter and discoloration throughout the three shifts (90.0%, 81.8%, and 84.4% respectively). All critical care nurses (100.0%) did not shake the bottle before using it during the morning shift and the vast majority of them did not follow this step during the evening and night shifts (100.0%, 93.9%, and 93.7% respectively), all critical care nurses (100.0%) throughout the three shifts diluted the propofol with D5W% if the dilution is necessary. None of critical care nurses discarded the unused portions and IV administration set after 12 hrs of propofol infusion.

Regarding ***midazolam***, all critical care nurses (100.0%) throughout the three shifts diluted the midazolam with D5W% or 0.9% NaCl if the dilution is necessary. Concerning ***diazepam***, all critical care nurses (100.0%) throughout the three shifts did not store the diazepam in a plastic syringe. From this table, it was found that there are no statistically significant differences between the three shifts in all items.

Table (15 - a): Distribution of critical care nurses' practices regarding sedatives dispensing

Dispensing	Morning						Evening						Night						Test of significance
	C/C		Inc/Inc		ND		C/C		Inc/Inc		ND		C/C		Inc/Inc		ND		
	No.	%	No.	%	No.	%	No.	%	No.	%	No.	%	No.	%	No.	%	No.	%	
Wash /disinfect hands	4	8.0	15	30.0	31	62.0	4	8.0	14	28.0	32	64.0	3	6.0	14	28.0	33	66.0	MCP=0.990
Wear clean gloves	23	46.0	0	0.0	27	54.0	21	42.0	0	0.0	29	58.0	22	44.0	0	0.0	28	56.0	X^2=0.16 P=0.922
Check prescribed sedative (first check)	50	100.0	0	0.0	0	0.0	50	100.0	0	0.0	0	0.0	50	100.0	0	0.0	0	0.0	-NA-
Read label on the drug container and check for expiration date (second check)	42	84.0	0	0.0	8	16.0	41	82.0	0	0.0	9	18.0	41	82.0	0	0.0	9	18.0	X^2=0.09 P=0.95
Compare sedative with physician's order	13	30.2	0	0.0	30	69.8	13	29.5	0	0.0	31	70.5	15	36.6	0	0.0	26	63.4	X^2=0.58 P=0.749
Avoid mixing sedatives with other drugs	28	100.0	0	0.0	0	0.0	33	100.0	0	0.0	0	0.0	31	100.0	0	0.0	0	0.0	-NA-
Maintain aseptic techniques during handling of sedatives	1	2.0	46	92.0	3	6.0	0	0.0	48	96.0	2	4.0	1	2.0	45	90.0	4	8.0	MCP=0.778

C / C: Correct or Complete   Inc / Inc: Incorrect or Incomplete   ND: Not done   NA: Not Applicable X^2: Chi-square test   MCP: Monte Carlo test

Table (15 - b): Distribution of critical care nurses' practices regarding specific sedatives dispensing

Dispensing	Morning						Evening						Night						Test of significance
	C/C		Inc/Inc		ND		C/C		Inc/Inc		ND		C/C		Inc/Inc		ND		
	No.	%	No.	%	No.	%	No.	%	No.	%	No.	%	No.	%	No.	%	No.	%	

Dispensing	Morning C/C No.	%	Inc/Inc No.	%	ND No.	%	Evening C/C No.	%	Inc/Inc No.	%	ND No.	%	Night C/C No.	%	Inc/Inc No.	%	ND No.	%	Test of significance
For propofol:																				
-Inspect bottle for particulate matter /discoloration	3	10.0	0	0.0	27	90.0	6	18.2	0	0.0	27	81.8	5	15.6	0	0.0	27	84.4	X²=0.87 P=0.648
- Shake the bottle well before use	0	0.0	0	0.0	30	100.0	2	6.1	0	0.0	31	93.9	2	6.3	0	0.0	30	93.7	MCP=0.452
-Dilute with D5W if dilution is necessary	27	100.0	0	0.0	0	0.0	31	100.0	0	0.0	0	0.0	29	100.0	0	0.0	0	0.0	-NA-
- Discard IV administration set after 12 hrs if administered directly from vial	0	0.0	0	0.0	23	100.0	0	0.0	0	0.0	27	100.0	0	0.0	0	0.0	26	100.0	-NA-
For midazolam:																				
- Diluted with D5W /0.9% NaCl if necessary.	1	100.0	0	0.0	0	0.0	2	100.0	0	0.0	0	0.0	1	100.0	0	0.0	0	0.0	-NA-
For diazepam:																				
- Avoid storing in plastic syringe	7	100.0	0	0.0	0	0.0	8	100.0	0	0.0	0	0.0	4	100.0	0	0.0	0	0.0	-NA-

C / C: Correct or Complete   Inc / Inc: Incorrect or Incomplete   ND: Not done   NA: Not Applicable   X²: Chi-square test   MCP: Monte Carlo test

(If number and percentage in any item is less than what is expected, this means that it is not applicable)

Table (16) shows the distribution of critical care nurses' practices regarding sedatives administration. It can be noted that all critical care nurses (100.0%) throughout the three shifts identified their patients correctly. Three quarters of critical care nurses (76.0%) assessed the IV site for presence of inflammation or vein irritation in the morning shift. While about two thirds of them did not assess the IV site in the evening and night shifts (68.0%, 64.0% respectively).The vast majority of critical care nurses (92.0%) ensured that the IV line is patent in the morning shift, while about three quarters of them followed this step in the evening and night shifts (78.0%, and 74.0% respectively). None of critical care nurses set the target level of sedation for their patients in collaboration with physician throughout the three shifts, and none of them titrated the sedatives according to sedation scale throughout the three shifts.

The majority of critical care nurses (84.0%) maintained the bed side rails elevated in the morning shift, and about two thirds of them followed this step in the evening and night shifts (70.0%, 68.0% respectively). All critical care nurses (100.0%) discarded disposable equipment correctly in the morning shift and about two thirds of them followed this step correctly in the evening and night shifts (84.0%, 86.0% respectively). The majority of critical care nurses (82.6%) removed the gloves after the administration of sedatives in the morning shift, and more than two thirds of them (71.4%) followed this step in the evening shift and about three fifths of them (59.1%) did it in the night shift. The majority of critical care nurses (82.0%) did not wash or disinfect their hands after the administration of sedatives in the night shift, and more than two thirds of them (68.0%) did not perform this in the evening shift and more than half of them (58.0%) did not follow it in the morning shift.

It can be noted from this table that there is a statistically significant differences between the three shifts in checking the IV site ($X2=23.72$, $P=0.0001$) and washing or disinfecting the hands ($X2=6.84$, $P=0.033$) while there are no statistically significant differences between the three shifts in the other items.

Table (16): Distribution of critical care nurses' practices regarding sedatives administration

Administration	Morning						Evening						Night						Test of significance
	C/C		Inc/Inc		ND		C/C		Inc/Inc		ND		C/C		Inc/Inc		ND		
	No.	%	No.	%	No.	%	No.	%	No.	%	No.	%	No.	%	No.	%	No.	%	
Check :- Patient identification	50	100.0	0	0.0	0	0.0	50	100.0	0	0.0	0	0.0	50	100.0	0	0.0	0	0.0	-NA-
- IV site for inflammation/ irritation	38	76.0	0	0.0	12	24.0	16	32.0	0	0.0	34	68.0	18	36.0	0	0.0	32	64.0	X^2=23.72 P=0.0001*
Ensure patency of IV line	46	92.0	0	0.0	4	8.0	39	78.0	0	0.0	11	22.0	37	74.0	0	0.0	13	26.0	X^2=5.88 P=0.053
Set target level of sedation in collaboration with physician	0	0.0	0	0.0	50	100.0	0	0.0	0	0.0	50	100.0	0	0.0	0	0.0	50	100.0	-NA-
Titrate sedatives according to sedation scale	0	0.0	0	0.0	50	100.0	0	0.0	0	0.0	50	100.0	0	0.0	0	0.0	50	100.0	-NA-
Maintain bed side rails elevated	42	84.0	0	0.0	8	16.0	35	70.0	0	0.0	15	30.0	34	68.0	0	0.0	16	32.0	X^2=3.95 P=0.139
Discard disposable equipment	50	100.0	0	0.0	0	0.0	42	84.0	6	12.0	2	4.0	43	86.0	5	10.0	2	4.0	MCp=0.075
Remove gloves	19	82.6	0	0.0	4	17.4	15	71.4	0	0.0	6	28.6	13	59.1	0	0.0	9	40.9	X^2=3.03 P=0.219
Wash /disinfect hands	0	0.0	21	42.0	29	58.0	0	0.0	16	32.0	34	68.0	0	0.0	9	18.0	41	82.0	X^2=6.84 P=0.033*

61

Administration	Morning						Evening						Night						Test of significance
	C/C		Inc/Inc		ND		C/C		Inc/Inc		ND		C/C		Inc/Inc		ND		
	No.	%	No.	%	No.	%	No.	%	No.	%	No.	%	No.	%	No.	%	No.	%	
	56.6±11.9 Mean± S.D =						46.2±15.3 Mean± S.D =						44.9±15.1 Mean± S.D =						
	49.2 ±10.9 Mean± S.D (average) =																		

C / C: Correct or Complete   Inc / Inc: Incorrect or Incomplete   ND: Not done   NA: Not Applicable

X^2: Chi-square test   MCP: Monte Carlo test   *: Statistically significant at $p \leq 0.05$

(If number and percentage in any item is less than what is expected, this means that it is not applicable)

62

Table (17) shows the distribution of critical care nurses' practices regarding implementation of non-pharmacological strategies. About two thirds of critical care nurses did not explain the procedure and its purpose(s) to their patients before sedatives administration in the morning and night shifts (65.9%, 70.3% respectively) and more than three quarters of them (76.2%) did not follow this strategy in the evening shift. More than two thirds of critical care nurses (68.3%) did not communicate clearly with their patients in the morning shift, and three quarters of them did not follow this strategy in the evening and night shifts (78.6%, 75.7% respectively).

The majority of critical care nurses did not provide verbal assurance to their patients throughout the three shifts (75.6%, 81.0%, and 83.8% respectively). About half of the critical care nurses allowed their patients to ventilate their anxiety and fear in the morning and night shifts (46.4%, 45.8% respectively). About half of critical care nurses (48.0%) did not adjust the light or control the noise in the morning shift, while slightly less than two thirds of them did not follow this strategy in the evening and night shifts (62.0%, 64.0% respectively).

From this table, it can be noted that there are no statistically significant differences between the three shifts in all items.

Table (17) : Distribution of critical care nurses' practices regarding implementation of non-pharmacological strategies

Non-pharmacological strategies	Morning						Evening						Night						Test of significance
	C/C		Inc/Inc		ND		C/C		Inc/Inc		ND		C/C		Inc/Inc		ND		
	No.	%	No.	%	No.	%	No.	%	No.	%	No.	%	No.	%	No.	%	No.	%	
Explain procedure to the patient	14	34.1	0	0.0	27	65.9	10	23.8	0	0.0	32	76.2	11	29.7	0	0.0	26	70.3	$X^2=1.08$ P=0.582
Communicate clearly with patient in quiet tone	13	31.7	0	0.0	28	68.3	9	21.4	0	0.0	33	78.6	9	24.3	0	0.0	28	75.7	$X^2=1.21$ P=0.547
Provide verbal assurance	10	24.4	0	0.0	31	75.6	8	19.0	0	0.0	34	81.0	6	16.2	0	0.0	31	83.8	$X^2=0.85$ P=0.654
Allow the patient to ventilate his anxiety/fear	13	46.4	0	0.0	15	53.6	10	38.5	0	0.0	16	61.5	11	45.8	0	0.0	13	54.2	$X^2=0.42$ P=0.811
Discuss with patient options available to alleviate the agitation	12	42.9	0	0.0	16	57.1	13	50.0	0	0.0	13	50.0	9	37.5	0	0.0	15	62.5	$X^2=0.8$ P=0.669
Adjust lighting and control the noise	3	6.0	23	46.0	24	48.0	3	6.0	16	32.0	31	62.0	2	4.0	16	32.0	32	64.0	MCp=0.502
	Mean± S.D = 18.2±21.9						Mean± S.D = 13.7±22.6						Mean± S.D = 12.9±22.4						
							Mean± S.D (average) = 14.9±17.7												

64

C / C: Correct or Complete   Inc / Inc: Incorrect or Incomplete   ND: Not done

X^2: Chi-square test   MCP: Monte Carlo test   *: Statistically significant at $p \leq 0.05$

(If number and percentage in any item is less than what is expected, this means that it is not applicable)

Table (18) shows the distribution of critical care nurses' practices regarding monitoring parameters before, during and after sedatives administration. It reveals that, none of critical care nurses monitored the *level of sedation* and the *level of pain* before, during or after sedatives administration throughout the three shifts. The majority of critical care nurses did not monitor the *level of consciousness* before sedatives administration throughout the three shifts (90.0%, 78.0% and 84.0% respectively), while about three quarters of them did not monitor LOC during sedatives administration throughout the three shifts (80.0%, 70.0% and 76.0% respectively), and about two thirds of them (73.0%, 62.1% and 62.5% respectively) did not monitor LOC after sedatives administration throughout the three shifts.

Regarding *respiratory rate*, more than three quarters of critical care nurses monitored the respiratory rate before and during sedatives administration in the morning shift (76.0%, 78.0% respectively) and about two thirds of them monitored the respiratory rate before and during sedatives administration in the evening and night shifts (63.3%, 62.0% respectively) and (68.0%, 66.0% respectively).

Regarding *oxygen saturation*, more than half of critical care nurses did not monitor the oxygen saturation before sedatives administration throughout the three shifts (52.0%, 55.1% , 56.0% respectively) and more than half of them did not monitor the oxygen saturation during sedatives administration throughout the three shifts (54.0%, 60.0% , 54.0% respectively), while more than three quarters of them (75.9%) monitored the oxygen saturation after sedatives administration in the evening shift, more than two thirds of them (66.7%) monitored the oxygen saturation after sedatives administration in the night shift and 56.8% of them monitored the oxygen saturation after sedatives administration in the morning shift.

Regarding *heart rate*, slightly less than three quarters of critical care nurses monitored the heart rate before sedatives administration in the morning and night shifts (72.0%, 72.0% respectively), and 64.0% of them monitored the heart rate in the evening shift. More than three quarters of critical care nurses (76.0%) monitored the heart rate during sedatives administration in the morning shift, and more than half of them monitored the heart rate during sedatives administration in the evening and night shifts (58.0%, 60.0%

respectively). Three quarters of critical care nurses (75.0%) monitored the heart rate after sedatives administration in the night shift, and more than half of them monitored the heart rate after sedatives administration in the morning and evening shifts (59.5%, 55.2% respectively).

Regarding **heart rhythm**, all critical care nurses (100.0%) did not monitor the heart rhythm before sedatives administration throughout the three shifts, and the majority of them did not monitor the heart rhythm during sedatives administration throughout the three shifts (86.0%, 86.0% and 90.0% respectively). Three quarters of critical care nurses (75.0%) monitored the heart rhythm after sedatives administration in the night shift, and more than half of them monitored it in the morning and evening shifts (59.5%, 55.2% respectively).

Regarding **blood pressure**, more than two thirds of critical care nurses monitored blood pressure before sedatives administration in the morning and night shifts (68.0%, 70.0% respectively), and 60.0% of them monitored it in the evening shift. More than three quarters of critical care nurses (76.0%) monitored blood pressure during sedatives administration in the morning shift, and more than half of them monitored it during sedatives administration in the evening and night shifts (54.0%, 56.0% respectively). Three quarters of critical care nurses (75.0%) monitored blood pressure after sedatives administration in the night shift, and more than half of them monitored it after sedatives administration in the morning and evening shifts (59.5%, 55.2% respectively).

Table (18): Distribution of critical care nurses' practices regarding monitoring parameters before, during and after sedatives administration

Monitoring parameters	Before sedatives administration (n=150)						During sedatives administration (n=150)						After sedatives administration (n=90)					
	Morning		Evening		Night		Morning		Evening		Night		Morning		Evening		Night	
	No.	%	No.	%	No.	%	No.	%	No.	%	No.	%	No.	%	No.	%	No.	%
Level of sedation																		
C/C	0	0.0	0	0.0	0	0.0	0	0.0	0	0.0	0	0.0	0	0.0	0	0.0	0	0.0
ND	50	100.0	50	100.0	50	100.0	50	100.0	50	100.0	50	100.0	37	100.0	29	100.0	24	100.0
Level of pain																		
C/C	0	0.0	0	0.0	0	0.0	0	0.0	0	0.0	0	0.0	0	0.0	0	0.0	0	0.0
ND	50	100.0	50	100.0	50	100.0	50	100.0	50	100.0	50	100.0	37	100.0	29	100.0	24	100.0
Level of consciousness																		
C/C	5	10.0	11	22.0	8	16.0	10	20.0	15	30.0	12	24.0	10	27.0	11	37.9	9	37.5
ND	45	90.0	39	78.0	42	84.0	40	80.0	35	70.0	38	76.0	27	73.0	18	62.1	15	62.5
Respiratory rate																		
C/C	38	76.0	31	63.3	34	68.0	39	78.0	31	62.0	33	66.0	22	59.5	16	55.2	18	75.0
ND	12	24.0	19	36.7	16	32.0	11	22.0	19	38.0	17	34.0	15	40.5	13	44.8	6	25.0
Oxygen saturation																		

Monitoring parameters	Before sedatives administration (n=150)						During sedatives administration (n=150)						After sedatives administration (n=90)					
	Morning		Evening		Night		Morning		Evening		Night		Morning		Evening		Night	
	No.	%	No.	%	No.	%	No.	%	No.	%	No.	%	No.	%	No.	%	No.	%
C/C	24	48.0	23	44.9	22	44.0	23	46.0	20	40.0	23	46.0	21	56.8	22	75.9	16	66.7
ND	26	52.0	27	55.1	28	56.0	27	54.0	30	60.0	27	54.0	16	43.2	7	24.1	8	33.3
Heart rate																		
C/C	36	72.0	32	64.0	36	72.0	38	76.0	29	58.0	30	60.0	22	59.5	16	55.2	18	75.0
ND	14	28.0	18	36.0	14	28.0	12	24.0	21	42.0	20	40.0	15	40.5	13	44.8	6	25.0
Heart rhythm																		
C/C	0	0.0	0	0.0	0	0.0	7	14.0	7	14.0	5	10.0	22	59.5	16	55.2	18	75.0
ND	9	100.0	9	100.0	5	100.0	43	86.0	43	86.0	45	90.0	15	40.5	13	44.8	6	25.0
Blood pressure																		
C/C	34	68.0	30	60.0	35	70.0	38	76.0	27	54.0	28	56.0	22	59.5	16	55.2	18	75.0
ND	16	32.0	20	40.0	15	30.0	12	24.0	23	46.0	22	44.0	15	40.5	13	44.8	6	25.0

C / C: Correct or Complete   ND: Not done   (If number and percentage in any item is less than what is expected, this means that it is not applicable)

Table (19) shows the distribution of critical care nurses' practices regarding documentation and reporting, in relation to **documentation**, none of critical care nurses documented pre-procedural assessment for the procedural sedation throughout the three shifts. About two thirds of critical care nurses completely documented drug's name, dose, route, time, date, flow rate throughout the morning and night shifts (58.0%, 64.0% respectively) and more than three quarters of them (76.0%) documented it in the evening shift. More than half of critical care nurses incompletely documented monitoring parameters in the morning and night shifts (58.0%, 56.0% respectively) and two thirds of them (66.0%) incompletely documented it in the evening shift. Three quarters of critical care nurses (75.0%) did not document adverse sedatives reactions in the evening shift, while two thirds of them (66.7%) did not document it in the morning shift and half of them (50.0%) did not document it in the night shift.

Regarding **reporting**, all critical care nurses (100.0%) reported adverse sedatives reactions to the physicians in the case of respiratory or cardiovascular adverse reactions throughout the three shifts. From this table, it was found that there are no statistically significant differences between the three shifts in all items.

Table (19): Distribution of critical care nurses' practices regarding documentation and reporting

Documentation and reporting	Morning						Evening						Night						Test of significance
	C/C		Inc/Inc		ND		C/C		Inc/Inc		ND		C/C		Inc/Inc		ND		
	No.	%	No.	%	No.	%	No.	%	No.	%	No.	%	No.	%	No.	%	No.	%	
Document:																			
• Pre-procedural assessment	0	0.0	0	0.0	11	100.0	0	0.0	0	0.0	10	100.0	0	0.0	0	0.0	13	100.0	-NA-
• Drug's name, dose, route, time, date, flow rate	29	58.0	13	26.0	8	16.0	38	76.0	5	10.0	7	14.0	32	64.0	7	14.0	11	22.0	$^{MC}p=0.169$
• Monitoring parameters	0	0.0	29	58.0	21	42.0	0	0.0	33	66.0	17	34.0	0	0.0	28	56.0	22	44.0	$X^2=1.17$ $p=0.558$
• dverse sedatives reactions	3	33.3	0	0.0	6	66.7	1	25.0	0	0.0	3	75.0	4	50.0	0	0.0	4	50.0	$^{MC}p=0.752$
Report:																			
• dverse sedative reactions: respiratory	4	100.0	0	0.0	0	0.0	2	100.0	0	0.0	0	0.0	6	100.0	0	0.0	0	0.0	-NA-
• Adverse sedative reactions: cardiovascular	5	100.0	0	0.0	0	0.0	2	100.0	0	0.0	0	0.0	2	100.0	0	0.0	0	0.0	-NA-
	Mean± S.D = 20.7±11.1						Mean± S.D = 20.0±14.1						Mean± S.D = 20.5±16.3						
	Mean± S.D (average) = 20.4±9.8																		

C / C: Correct or Complete   Inc / Inc: Incorrect or Incomplete   ND: Not done   NA: Not Applicable

X^2: Chi-square test ^{MC}p: Monte Carlo test   *: Statistically significant at p ≤ 0.05

(If number and percentage in any item is less than what is expected, this means that it is not applicable)

Table (20) shows distribution of critical care nurses according to mean percentage of practices regarding safe use of sedatives. It was found that critical care nurses had a good level of practices in relation to sedatives drugs administration by syringe pump and IV bolus injections, while critical care nurses had poor level of practices in relation to sedative drugs prescription, dispensing, administration, drip infusion, none pharmacological strategy, monitoring and documentation and reporting.

Table (20): Distribution of critical care nurses according to mean percentage of practices regarding safe use of sedatives

Practices	Shifts			
	Morning	**Evening**	**Night**	**Average**
• *Prescribing*	22.4±17.1	21.6±14.9	20.7±15.6	21.6±12.0
• *Dispensing*	32.8±10.1	34.5±11.6	33.2±11.7	33.5±8.6
• *Administering*	56.6±11.9	46.2±15.3	44.9±15.1	49.2 ±10.9
- *Continuous IV infusion by Syringe pump (appendix iv)*	87.4±7.3	77.6±28.0	88.9±7.4	83.9±20.9
- *Continuous IV Drip infusion (appendix iv)*	71.1±15.3	73.4±13.9	42.6±32.3	48.7±29.7
- *Intermittent IV Bolus injection (appendix iv)*	80.6±5.6	78.0±18.0	82.6±7.5	79.1±15.4
- *Non-pharmacological strategies*	18.2±21.9	13.7±22.6	12.9±22.4	14.9±17.7
• *Monitoring*	34.2±13.2	29.4±15.3	30.3±15.7	31.3±9.3
• *Documenting and reporting*	20.7±11.1	20.0±14.1	20.5±16.3	20.4±9.8
Total practice	37.7±6.7	34.7±7.9	33.8±8.3	35.4±5.9

Good = ≥75% of total score   Fair = between 50% to less than 75% of total score   Poor = < 50% of total score

Part 6: Relationship between critical care nurses knowledge and practices regarding safe use of sedatives and their characteristics

Table (21) shows the total mean percentage score of critical care nurses' knowledge and practices regarding safe use of sedatives. Concerning **nurses' knowledge**, this table represents that, the mean knowledge score was 50.6±6.7, and the minimum score was 38.1 and the maximum score was 71.4. More than half of critical care nurses (58.0%) had poor level of knowledge, and 42.0% of them had fair level of knowledge. Regarding **nurses' practices**, the mean practices score was 35.4±5.9, and the minimum score was 21.9 and the maximum score was 51.5. The vast majority of critical care nurses (96.0%) had poor level of practices; while only 4.0% of them had fair level of practices. There is no correlation and no statistically significant differences between the total mean percentage score of knowledge and practices (r = 0.105, p = 0.468).

Table (21): Total mean percentage score of critical care nurses' knowledge and practices regarding safe use of sedatives

Level of knowledge and practices	Knowledge		Practices		Pearson correlation coefficient (r)
	No.	Total mean percentage score	No.	Total mean percentage score	
Good	0	0.0	0	0.0	
Fair	21	42.0%	2	4.0%	r = 0.105, p = 0.468
Poor	29	58.0%	48	96.0%	
Mean ±SD	50.6±6.7		35.4±5.9		
Min-Max	38.1-71.4		21.9-51.5		

Good = ≥75% of total score   Fair = between 50% to less than 75% of total score   Poor = < 50% of total score

*: Statistically significant at p ≤ 0.05

73

Table (22) illustrates the total mean percentage score of critical care nurses' knowledge and practices regarding safe use of sedatives according to their characteristics. *Regarding the sex*, female nurses had higher level of knowledge (mean=51.2±7.9) than male nurses (mean=49.7±4.5), while the level of practices was higher in male nurses (mean=36.0±6.9) than female nurses (mean=34.9±5.3). *Regarding the level of education*, nurses who hold diploma degree had higher level of knowledge (mean=52.8±9.1) than nurses who hold bachelor degree (mean=49.9±5.7), while the level of practices was higher in nurses who hold bachelor degree (mean=35.5±5.8) than nurses who hold diploma degree (mean=35.0±6.7). *Regarding the ICU,* the level of knowledge and practices was higher in nurses who are working in general ICU (mean=50.9±5.5, mean=35.5±5.4) than nurses who are working in casualty ICU (mean=50.3±7.6, mean=35.3±6.5).

Regarding **experience in ICU**, nurses who have experience 5<10 years had higher level of knowledge (mean=55.2±9.2) than nurses who have experience 1< 5 years (mean=46.0±2.3) and nurses who have experience less than one year (mean=50.6±5.9), while the level of practices was higher in nurses who have experience less than one year (mean=35.5±5.2) than nurses who have experience 5<10 years (mean=35.3±7.6), and nurses who have experience 1< 5 years (mean=35.2±7.5).

From this table, it can be noted that there is a statistically significant differences between the level of knowledge and nurses' experience (F=4.903, p=0.012*), while there are no statistically significant differences between the level of knowledge and level of practices regarding critical care nurses' sex, level of education and ICUs.

Table (22): The total mean percentage score of critical care nurses' knowledge and practices regarding safe use of sedatives according to their characteristics

Critical care nurses' characteristics		N=50	Knowledge score	Significance	Practices score	Significance
• Sex	Male	21	49.7±4.5	t=0.776	36.0±6.9	t=0.604
	Female	29	51.2±7.9	P=0.442	34.9±5.3	P=0.549
• Educational level	Bachelor degree	38	49.9±5.7	t=1.301	35.5±5.8	t=0.269
	Diploma degree	12	52.8±9.1	P=0.199	35.0±6.7	P=0.789
• ICU	Casualty ICU (unit I)	27	50.3±7.6	t=0.314	35.3±6.5	t=0.084
	General ICU (unit III)	23	50.9±5.5	P=0.755	35.5±5.4	P=0.933
• ICU experience (years)	Less than 1	32	50.6±5.9	F=4.903	35.5±5.2	F=0.008
	1< 5	9	46.0±2.3	P=0.012*	35.2±7.5	P=0.992
	5 < 10	9	55.2±9.2		35.3±7.6	

t: t-test   F: ANOVA test   *: Statistically significant at p ≤ 0.05

Chapter V

Discussion

Discussion

Sedation management in the ICU is primarily the purview of the bedside staff nurses. The depth of sedation is prescribed by doctors; observed and recorded by the nursing staff as they are responsible for titrating the drugs infused and monitoring their effects. Thus, In order to achieve effective and safe sedative management, the knowledge and practices of critical care nurses about sedative drugs should be assessed. Young et al (2000) [28] concluded that to enable effective sedation, nurses require knowledge and skills to provide the beneficial effects of sedation and avoid both over and under sedation. Guttormsona et al (2010) [118] emphasized that the nurses' knowledge regarding sedatives and their management is an important area of future research and should be evaluated. Therefore, this study was conducted to identify critical care nurses' knowledge and practices regarding the safe use of sedatives.

The findings of the present study show that the level of nurses' knowledge regarding safe use of sedatives was generally fair. This lack of knowledge may be due to lack of focus on sedative drugs and sedation assessment during the undergraduate courses, absence of teaching materials about sedation in the hospital, absence of pre-employment orientation programs, in-service education and training programs regarding sedation assessment and management in the hospital. Moreover, lack of time for independent self learning, in addition to nurses' exhaustion and burnout due to work load or due to the working in more than one hospital which may hinder their ability to read and update their knowledge.

In this respect, Walker et al (2006) [18] recommended that induction of education programs about sedation therapy should be in place for all critical care nurses in intensive care units. This aims to develop knowledge, skills and confidence to improve decision-making in relation to sedation management at the bedside. Furthermore, El-Shenawi S (2002) [119] recommended that a library should be available in the hospital with up to date scientific journals and books to promote self learning. However, the results of the present study stands in opposition with Mehta et al (2007) [120] results, which revealed that nurses' knowledge about sedation was very good.

The findings of the present study demonstrate that the critical care nurses' practices regarding sedatives were generally poor. This may be due to combination of several factors, some were related to the hospital system, and the others were related to critical care nurses themselves. This poor score could be due to absence of written sedation protocol or guidelines and sedation scales in ICUs guiding sedative administration, insufficient information to deal with sedatives, inadequate supervision by the nurses' supervisors, lack of communication and collaboration between nursing staff and medical staff in determining patients' sedation needs, and high workload.

In relation to nurses' experience, it was found that there is a significant relationship between nurses' knowledge and their experience. This study shows that nurses with more experience had higher level of knowledge than those with less experience. This knowledge may be developed through the experience and acquired from clinical practice or nurses' self learning. Egerod et al (2002) [97], and Walker et al (2006) [18] found that the more experienced nurses provide a better quality of sedation, use less sedatives, and are more able to articulate their decision-making than less experienced nurses. Also, Egerod et al (2002) [97] found that experienced nurses look for other causes of agitation prior to administering sedatives, while inexperienced nurses use sedatives more readily.

The findings of the present study demonstrate that critical care nurses did not use a written sedation protocol, policy or guidelines. This is mainly related to absence of sedation protocol in ICU, and due to the low awareness of the fact that the sedatives are high alert medications and require special attention and extra care when dealing with it in critical care settings. These findings are in opposition with findings of other studies which indicated that sedation protocol is used in more than half of ICUs in Australia and Germany [121, 122], in about two thirds of ICUs in United States [123] and in more than three quarters of ICUs in United Kingdom [124].

Weir et al (2008) [125] concluded that to ensure safe sedation management of critically ill patients, all members of the health care team within the ICUs need further encouragement and teaching sessions to convince them of the benefits of using a scoring tool and clinical guidelines. Slomka et al (2000) [98] suggested that protocols could be a learning tool and aid in decision making especially among junior staff by increasing knowledge and confidence and facilitating decision-making at the bedside. Quality assurance studies have shown that incorporation of a sedation protocol and scale into routine practice can reduce the incidence of oversedation, the duration of mechanical ventilation, and ICU length of stay [14, 126].

The current study demonstrates that about half of the sedated critically ill patients were sedated adequately. These results indicate the importance of introducing sedation protocol and sedation scale into clinical practice which enables critical care nurses to manage sedation adequately and to play a key role in providing safe and effective care to the sedated critically ill patients.

The findings of present study illustrate that the majority of sedated critically ill patients were attached to mechanical ventilation. There are many reasons why a patient attached to mechanical ventilator needs to be sedated. Being in the ICU on a ventilator can be very anxiety provoking. Mechanically ventilated patients need sedation to facilitate tolerance of endotracheal tube and to induce amnesia. These results are in the line with another study conducted by Samuelson et al (2003) [127] who found that the vast majority of mechanically ventilated patients were routinely sedated in ICUs. Ba-alwi A (2008) [25] found that about half of critically ill patients were sedated.

The present study reveals that the most common indication to sedate critically ill patients is to decrease their anxiety and agitation. This is mainly because critically ill patients are often scared, isolated and aware that they are in a life-threatening situation and often cannot adequately communicate their feelings [34]. Furthermore, critically ill patients often require invasive, painful or distressing treatment for days, and so need to be able to tolerate these therapies. Studies [97, 128] have shown that about half of patients in ICU exhibit anxiety and more than two thirds of them demonstrate agitated behavior.

79

The options for sedation in the ICU are limited, with benzodiazepines and propofol being the most commonly used agents [4, 51, 129, 130]. *The findings of the present study demonstrate that* the most commonly used sedatives in intensive care units are propofol, midazolam and diazepam. These findings are in the line with another study conducted by Murdoch et al (2000) [131] which revealed that the propofol is the most widely used ICU sedative. Also, O'Connor et al (2010) [121] found that for sedation, midazolam and propofol were equally used (approximately 50% each).

In relation to sedatives prescription, the present study demonstrates that critical care nurses practices in relation to checking the prescription orders was poor. These may be due to incomplete or unclear orders or because nurses frequently administer medications, it may appear to be a routine activity. El-Sayed M (2012) [132] found that nurses mentioned illegibility (unclear hand writing of physician) and the confusing order/instruction as a main sources of error. Also, El-Sayed M (2012) [132] found that in relation to the prescribing stage, about one quarter of sources of medication adverse drug events (MAEs) were in these stage.

Randen et al (2010) [128] found that two thirds of the nurses reported that they did not find what they needed in the documentation to give adequate sedation. Another study conducted by Walker et al (2006) [18] concluded that prescriptions of sedation based on explicit goals of sedation therapy and optimum levels of sedation linked to a score may improve clarity for the nurses at the bedside and reduce variability in decision-making between nurses with different levels of confidence and experience. Tanios et al (2009) [123] found that over two-thirds of respondents agreed or strongly agreed that physicians considered their assessments when ordering sedation and that sedation orders were written with broad parameters for nurses discretion. Weinert et al (2001) [133] found that physicians often do not clearly document the sedation goals, which may fluctuate with the patient's condition.

The practice of checking the patient's chart for allergies continues to be a basic and integral process of safe medication administration, determining whether a patient has allergies before administering medication is fundamental to nursing practice [134]. *The present study shows that the majority of critical care nurses didn't check the patient medical condition and history including current medication and allergies.* This may be due to the insufficient information regarding sedative drugs, incomplete recording of pertinent health or drug information on patient's chart and inadequate nurses' supervision and workload.

In relation to sedatives dispensing, the present study shows that the majority of critical care nurses practices in relation to hand washing before and after sedatives handling were poor. Hand washing is frequently forgotten or inadequate; several factors may contribute to this including lack of adequate hand washing equipment and supplies, insufficient time to accomplish hand washing, high workload, health habit, lack of role model, lack of close guidance and supervision by senior staff, and concern about repeated hand washing has on the condition of the skin.

The current study also indicates that the nurses replace the hand washing by wearing the gloves. These findings are in the line with other findings of El-Shenawi S (2002) [119], who indicated that the majority of nurses often omit washing when gloves are worn. This may be attributed to the fact that nurses believe that gloves provide enough protection to keep hands clean. It is very important to wash hands after removing gloves, gloving doesn't replace hand washing for many reasons; gloves may be punctured or leak, organisms on hands can multiply rapidly inside the warm moist environment of the gloves.

Also, it can be noted from the findings of this study that the majority of critical care nurses double check the sedatives during dispensing. Double-checks have been reported to have a significant effect on reduction of the incident rate of dispensing errors [96]. This finding stands in opposition with El-Sayed M (2012) [132] findings, which revealed that none of nurses double check the regular or high alert medications. *In this study, it was noted that the majority of critical care nurses had poor score in specific sedatives dispensing.* This may be due to insufficient nurses' information regarding sedatives special precautions and absence of instruction about the use of these drugs on the patient's chart, in addition to nurses' unawareness of importance of reading the instructions written on drug ampoule especially for propofol.

In relation to the administration stage, the present study demonstrates the absence of collaboration between critical care nurses and physicians in determining the appropriate target level of sedation. These findings stand in opposition with Randen et al (2010) [128] findings, which revealed that the majority of nurses stated that the most important variable in assessing sedation needs is the collaboration between the nurses and physicians. Furthermore, Randen et al (2010) [128] found that most nurses perceived that decision-making about sedation levels was made in collaboration with physicians. Agreement about sedation goals has been reported as important by nurses in other studies [17, 130]. Tanios et al (2009) [123] found that three fifths of respondents agreed that sedation goals were clearly communicated between physicians and nurses. Weinert et al (2001) [133] found that physicians communicate with nurses about issues related to sedation through several mechanisms: bedside visits, telephone updates, and sedative medication orders. In this respect, Gaber M (2010) [135] recommended that the separation between the physicians and nurses should be reduced during the nurses' undergraduate and postgraduate education.

Mehta S (2007) [120] found that nurses believes that they are generally better able to evaluate patients' sedation needs as compared with physicians, who, because they see the patients less frequently, may not appreciate their sedation requirements and thus order inadequate doses. Also this is supported by Weinert et al (2001) [133] who found that when nurses and physicians do not discuss their different priorities for sedation, misinterpretation is likely. Nurses think that their ability to continually evaluate a patient's need for sedation and response to medications is an advantage compared with the situation of physicians who observe the patient's behavior only intermittently or who are temporarily covering for the primary physician. However, nurses think they are disadvantaged in managing sedative therapy if they are not informed about the patient's medical status such as proximity to weaning.

Furthermore, it was noted that there was no communication between critical care nurses during the handover regarding the appropriate and the current level of sedation. This mainly related to the absence of using sedation scale and low awareness regarding the risks of oversedation and undersedation. Nursing staff with varying degrees of expertise will change several times over the working day. Therefore, sedation level should be communicated during nursing handover. In this respect, Walker et al (2006) [18] found that the vast majority of nurses agreed that the patient's sedation score should be communicated during handover of the bedside nurse at the shift change. Also, Westcott C (1995) [136] concluded that the use of a sedation score will promote continuity of care.

The present study shows that none of the critical care nurses titrate sedative drugs. This can be related mainly to lack of awareness that titration of sedatives is one of the main responsibilities of critical care nurses, in addition to absence of sedation scale that allows sedatives to be titrated appropriately. These results are in contrast with results of other studies [97, 98] which demonstrated that the nurses manage the dose and frequency of sedation by titrating sedation within prescribed limits, to achieve the agreed target level. Furthermore, Walker et al (2006) [18] found that nurses reported that they play a key role in the continual assessment of patients' need of sedation, as well as determining the dosage and frequency in titrating sedatives within prescribed limits.

The findings of the present study demonstrate that about two thirds of sedatives were administered by continuous IV infusions. Continuous IV infusions are very frequently used for the following reasons. First, many patients have difficulty communicating their sedatives requirement because of the presence of an endotracheal tube or altered level of consciousness. Second, continuous IV infusion offers a more consistent level of sedation that may improve patient comfort compared with intermittent bolus dosing [137]. Third, continuous IV sedation frees the nurses' time to address multiple issues. This finding is in the line with the findings of another study conducted by Salgado et al (2010) [138] who found that sedative drugs were predominantly administered by continuous infusion for the majority of sedated patients, while the intermittent IV bolus was used only for less than one fifth of sedated patients.

However, for methods of continuous IV infusion delivery, the results of this study show that more than half of continuous IV sedatives were given via drip infusion. Administration of sedatives via drip involves high risk to patients because of the difficulties in controlling the flow rate over 24 hours which can lead to oversedation or undersedation and its associated complications. The causes of these wrong practices are mainly related to lack of adequate education about the risks of oversedation or undersedation and insufficient number of functioning syringe pumps.

However, intermittent IV bolus injection was used mainly for the control of anxiety and agitation, and during procedural sedation. On the same line, a study conducted by Salgado et al (2010) [138] reported that intermittent IV bolus sedation was used for the treatment of withdrawal syndrome, control of severe agitation, short-term procedures and in the postoperative period.

The present study demonstrates that the majority of the critical care nurses have achieved a low score in implementing non-pharmacological strategies to their patients'. This can be explained by the fact that critical care nurses tend to focus on technological or physical care for their patients rather than psychological aspects, in addition to lack of nurses' education regarding non-pharmacological strategies, communication difficulties with the patients, lack of nurses' experience, and high workload. These results are supported by Aboud R (2008) [139] study, which revealed that nurses did not have the essential communication skills, and nurses learned subconsciously that minimizing interactions with patients may reduce their own anxiety, and as a result, patients will suffer from repetition of failure trials of communication. In this respect, Weinert et al (2001) [133] found that critical care nurses thought that non-pharmacological strategies alleviating patients' anxiety or behavior (through close physical presence, attempts at communication and reassurance) is time-consuming, is often ineffective, and interferes with a nurse's ability to carry out more immediate life-supporting activities. On the contrary, Peck et al (2009) [77] emphasized that the non-pharmacological techniques should always be explored to reduce the use of sedatives.

In relation to the monitoring stage, the present study reveals that none of critical care nurses assessed or monitored the level of sedation using sedation scale. This can be related to many reasons including absence of sedation protocols or policy to use sedation scale, lack of awareness that sedation assessment is the main responsibilities of nursing staff, absence of item regarding sedation in the nursing record such as sedation scale, lack of supervision from senior staff, in addition to excessive workload. The findings, however, are inconsistent with another study conducted by Reschreiter et al (2008) [124] who found that the majority of ICUs use sedation scales. Ramsay et al (2000) [140] stated that sedation scale should be the sixth vital signs. If the sedation level was assessed with the same zeal as other vital signs are, it would have better chance of being treated properly.

The present study demonstrates that none of critical care nurses' assessed or monitored the level of pain in sedated critically ill patients. This can be explained by the lack of supervision from senior staff, absence of items related to pain in the nursing record. In this respect, Abd El-Razak M (2005) [141] recommended that the pain should be considered the fifth vital signs. This is supported with many studies which argued that pain should be considered to be the fifth vital signs and be measured and documented as carefully and regularly as heart rate, blood pressure, respiratory rate and temperature [142, 143].

Also it was noted in this study that critical care nurses rely on the vital signs to assess the level of sedation, in addition; about half of them reported using vital signs to determine the level of sedation. These results are in the line with Samuelson et al (2003) [127] results, which revealed that only less than one fifth of ICUs used sedation scales, while the remaining four fifths described a variety of means such as vital signs, facial expression, tolerance to ventilation and level of consciousness as methods for assessing sedation. Furthermore, Randen et al (2010) [128] found that more than half of critical care nurses stated that they use Glasgow coma scale in their personal sedation practice.

The sedation guidelines (2002) [4] state that, "vital signs such as blood pressure and heart rate are not specific or sensitive markers of the level of sedation among critically ill patients". The published report from the consensus conference on sedation assessment (AACN & Abbott Laboratories, 2004) [6] indicates that vital signs are assessed under the heading of hemodynamic stability and that the goal of maintaining hemodynamic stability falls under the more global concept of maintaining physiological stability. Within this consensus statement, a stated goal of sedation is to maintain physiological stability. This implies that vital signs may be used to define endpoints for hemodynamic stability and should be routinely assessed during periods of sedation [29].

The findings of the present study demonstrate that critical care nurses practices regarding documentation and reporting was poor. This can be explained by the fact that the present nursing record didn't contain items related to sedation scale or sedation management, in addition to the lack of supervision from the senior staff. Randen et al (2010) [128] found that nurses reported that routine documentation of sedation levels was fairly common. Using of sedation scale may improve accurate documentation and facilitate communication between ICU caregivers [1].

A fundamental element of nursing care in ICU is providing optimal comfort to patients. The technological nature of the ICU is stressful for both staff and patients and sedation is important to maintain comfort and reduce their risk of harm [21]. Therefore, critical care nurses require not only an extensive knowledge and training regarding safe sedatives use, but also an understanding of what is happening to the critically ill patient and the impact of the sedative will have on that patient [21, 136].

Chapter VI

Conclusion

&Recommendations

Conclusion & Recommendations

Conclusion

The present study highlights the critical care nurses' knowledge and practices regarding the safe use of sedatives. Based on the results of this study, it can be concluded that:

In relation to *critical care nurses' knowledge*, the findings of the present study shows that the level of nurses' knowledge regarding safe use of sedatives was generally fair. Regarding to *critical care nurses' practices*, the results of the current study demonstrates that the level of nurses' practices regarding safe use of sedatives was generally poor.

Recommendations

Based on the findings of the current study, the following recommendations can be suggested:

Educational recommendations:
- Increase the focus on sedative drugs, sedation assessment and safe use of sedatives during the undergraduate courses to equip the students with the necessary knowledge and skills that enable them to use sedatives safely later on.
- Pre-employment orientation, in-service education and training programs about sedation assessment and management should be conducted for critical care nurses with collaboration of educational institutes to raise their awareness regarding safe use of sedatives.
- Learning facilities such as up to date scientific journals and books , posters , and results of researches , in addition to access to internet should be available in the hospitals to promote self learning regarding safe use of sedative

Practical recommendations:
- Introducing both subjective & objective sedation scales into clinical practice and training all critical care nurses about how using them.
- Sedation level should be systemically assessed at regular intervals, using both subjective and objective scales.

- Sedatives should be titrated according to sedation scale.

- Team approach should be considered in the care of sedated critically ill patients to allow critical care nurses' participation in sedation management decision.

Administrative recommendations:

- Local sedation guidelines or protocol should be available in a written form at the ICUs to be followed by critical care nurses and other health care providers.

- Critical care nurses and intern nurses should be instructed & supervised by their supervisors and preceptors regarding the use of sedation scales and implementation of the sedation guidelines or protocol.

- Integrating sedation scales into the routine assessment format or the assessment flow sheet of the critically ill patients.

- Hospital budget should be directed to provide the needed equipment for sedation level determination such as bispectral index monitor and to provide sufficient number of functioning syringe pumps for continuous IV sedative infusion.

Research related recommendation:

- Consider further studies about sedatives and sedation management in different areas such as:
  - Exploring the effect of using daily interruption of continuous sedative infusion on the duration of mechanical ventilation and length of ICU stay.
  - Exploring factors influencing critical care nurses' sedation practices.
  - Measuring the effectiveness of using sedation scale and protocol on critically ill patients' outcomes.

- Consider replication of the current study on a larger sample size for generalization of results.

Chapter VII

Summary

Summary

Management of sedation during critical illness has been a focus of increased interest, particularly over the past decade. Administration of sedative drugs is often considered to be a standard part of the routine care of critically ill patients. Patients admitted to the ICU receive sedation for many hours and even days, largely because of their dependence on mechanical ventilation, poor general condition, high treatment and monitoring invasiveness, nursing maneuvers, and many other factors such as isolation, sleep deprivation and communication impairment. Therefore, sedation is crucial to the management of critically ill patients. Adequate sedation hinders the reaction to stress, prevents anxiety, increases comfort, and improves tolerance to endotracheal intubation and mechanical ventilation, thus facilitating nursing work [76, 138, 144].

The safe and effective use of sedatives must be an integral part of intensive care practice. The most important aspect of ICU sedation is understanding of the drugs given to patients and their specific advantages and disadvantages. Each drug is ideal for a specific use. Therefore, management of sedation in the critically ill patient requires knowledge, skills and a thorough understanding of the sedation process, a lack thereof can have catastrophic outcomes [89].

Critical care nurse has a major role in the management of sedation; it is a part of the nurses' role to manage sedation therapy according to patients' needs and avoid complications of over and under sedation. One of the obstacles for providing appropriate education to critical care nurses and thereby improving patients' care is the lack of information regarding the current knowledge and practices of critical care nurses working in ICU. Therefore, this study was conducted to identify critical care nurses' knowledge and practices regarding the safe use of sedatives. This study reflects what is really done in ICUs, points out gaps between actual practices and current recommendations and international guidelines, and could serve as a basis for the elaboration of national guidelines [18].

This study was conducted at the casualty intensive care unit (Unit I) and the general intensive care unit (Unit III) at the Alexandria Main University Hospital. A convenient sample of fifty critical care nurses including technical and intern nurses who were involved in providing direct patient care throughout the three different shifts (morning, evening and night) in the previously mentioned units were included in this study.

To accomplish the aim of the current study; two tools were used for data collection. Tool one *"safe use of sedatives observation checklist"* and tool two *"safe use of sedatives structured questionnaire"*. Both tools were developed by the researcher after reviewing the related literature [4, 34, 55, 68, 90, 96, 110, 114-117].

An official letter was directed from the Faculty of Nursing in Alexandria University to hospital administrative authority in order to obtain their acceptance to collect the necessary data from the selected ICUs. Safe use of sedatives structured questionnaire (Tool II) was developed in Arabic by the researcher based on reviewing the related literature. Both tools of the study were tested for content validity by seven experts in the fields of critical care nursing and pharmacology. Accordingly; all necessary modifications were done.

The researcher explained the objectives of the study to critical care nurses. Voluntary participation and right to refuse to participate in the study were emphasized. A pilot study was conducted on ten critical care nurses to test the clarity, applicability and feasibility of the developed tools; and the data were excluded from the total sample. Safe use of sedatives structured questionnaire (Tool II) was tested for its reliability by using Cronbach's coefficient alpha and the reliability was 0.72 which is acceptable.

The data was collected as follows:

• Safe use of sedatives observation checklist (Tool I) was used to assess critical care nurse's practices regarding the safe use of sedatives. Each nurse involved in providing direct patient care was observed by the researcher during use of sedatives three times over the different three shifts (morning, evening and night) once during each shift.

• After finishing all observations, safe use of sedatives structured questionnaire (Tool II) was distributed to the critical care nurses who were observed during use of sedatives to assess their knowledge in relation to safe use of sedatives. Critical care nurses were asked to answer the questionnaire and to bring it back to the researcher at the end of the shift. The researcher was available to clarify any question.

- Data were collected by the researcher during approximately three months over starting from 10th of January 2012 to 5th of April 2012.

Results of the study:

It was found in this study that more than half of critical care nurses are females and the majority of them are less than 25 years. Concerning the level of education, it was found that more than three quarters of critical care nurses hold a bachelor degree of nursing, and the rest of them hold a diploma degree.

In relation to job-related data of critical care nurses, more than half of critical care nurses were working in casually care unit and the rest of them in general ICU. Regarding their job title, three quarters of critical care nurses were intern nurses, and the rest of them are technical nurses. Regarding the duration of nursing experience in ICU, it was found that slightly less than two thirds of critical care nurses have an experience in ICUs less than one year.

Concerning critical care nurses' knowledge, the findings of the present study shows that the level of nurses' knowledge regarding safe use of sedatives was generally fair. In relation to critical care nurses' practices, the findings of the current study demonstrates that critical care nurses' practices regarding safe use of sedatives were generally poor.

Also, it was noticed that all critical care nurses didn't use any sedation scale or pain scale to assess the level of sedation and the level of pain. Furthermore, critical care nurses did not follow sedation protocol or guidelines.

It was found that there is a significant relationship between nurses' knowledge and their experience, critical care nurses with more experience have higher level of knowledge (mean= 55.2±9.2) than those with less experience.

The most common indications to sedate critically ill patients were to reduce their anxiety and agitation, facilitate tolerance of endotracheal tube and to increase patients' tolerance for procedures. The most frequently used sedatives were propofol, midazolam and diazepam.

Also, it was found that about half of the sedated critically ill patients were sedated adequately, while the rest of them were either over sedated or under sedated.

The results of this study provide several insights that may help to improve our clinical practice and to draw up national guidelines for sedatives practices. Critical care nurses need more knowledge and skills in relation to safe use of sedatives.   Clearly, efforts should be directed to elaborate appropriate protocol/ guidelines in the ICU to facilitate the regular use of sedation scales, and to ensure the safe use of sedatives. Such efforts could result in a vast improvement in patient comfort and clinical outcomes.

Based on the findings of this study it can be recommended that:

- Increase the focus on sedative drugs, sedation assessment and safe use of sedatives during the undergraduate courses to equip the students with the necessary knowledge and skills that enable them to use sedatives safely later on.

- Pre-employment orientation, in-service education and training programs about sedation assessment and management should be conducted for critical care nurses with collaboration of educational institutes to raise their awareness regarding safe use of sedatives.
- Learning facilities such as up to date scientific journals and books , posters , and results of researches, in addition to access to internet should be available in the hospitals to promote self learning regarding safe use of sedative
- Introducing both subjective & objective sedation scales into clinical practice and training all critical care nurses about how using them.
- Sedation level should be systemically assessed at regular intervals, using both subjective and objective scales and should be considered the sixth vital signs.
- Sedatives should be titrated according to sedation scale.

- Team approach should be considered in the care of sedated critically ill patients to allow critical care nurses' participation in sedation management decision.

- Local sedation guidelines or protocol should be available in a written form at the ICUs to be followed by critical care nurses and other health care providers.

- Critical care nurses and intern nurses should be instructed & supervised by their supervisors and preceptors regarding the use of sedation scales and implementation of the sedation guidelines or protocol.

- Integrating sedation scales into the routine assessment format or the assessment flow sheet of the critically ill patients.

- Hospital budget should be directed to provide the needed equipment for sedation level determination such as bispectral index monitor and to provide sufficient number of functioning syringe pumps for continuous IV sedative infusion.

- Consider further studies about sedatives and sedation management in different areas such as:
  o Exploring the effect of using daily interruption of continuous sedative infusion on the duration of mechanical ventilation and length of ICU stay.
  o Exploring factors influencing critical care nurses' sedation practices.
  o Measuring the effectiveness of using sedation scale and protocol on critically ill patients' outcomes.
- Consider replication of the current study on a larger sample size for generalization of results.

Chapter VIII

References

References

1.   Devlin J, Fraser G, Kanji S, Riker R. Sedation assessment in critically ill adults. The Annals of Pharmacotherapy. 2001; 35 (12): 1624-32.

2. Ebert T. Special case report: Current strategies in ICU sedation. Anesthesiology News and Pharmacy Practice. 2001. Available at: http://www. dexmedetomidine.com%2F114SRfinal.pdf. Retrieved on: 28/4/2012.

3.   Peruzzi W, Hurt K. Approach to sedation in the ICU. Journal of Critical Care. 2005; 24 (1):27-33

4.   Jacobi J, Fraser G, Coursin D, Riker R, Fontaine D, Wittbrodt E, Chalfin D, Masica M, Bjerke H, Coplin W, Crippen D, Fuchs B, Kelleher R, Marik P, Nasraway S, Murray M, Peruzzi W, Lumb P. Clinical practice guidelines for the sustained use of sedatives and analgesics in the critically ill adult. Critical Care Med. 2002; 30(1): 119-41.

5. Mehta S, Burry L, Fischer S, Martinez J, Hallett D, Bowman D, Wong C, Meade M, Stewart T, Cook D. Canadian survey of the use of sedatives, analgesics, and neuromuscular blocking agents in critically ill patients. Critical Care Medicine. 2006; 34(2):374-80.

6. Abbott Laboratories. American Association of Critical-Care Nurses, Saint Thomas Health System Sedation Expert Panel Members. Consensus conference on sedation assessment: A collaborative venture. Critical Care Nurse. 2004; 24(2):33-41.

7.   Kaplan L, Bailey H. Bispectral index (BIS) monitoring of ICU patients on continuous infusions of sedatives and paralytics reduces sedative drug utilization and cost. Critical Care Nurse. 2000;4 (Suppl 1): S110

8.   Kress J, Pohlman A, O'Connor M, Hall J. Daily interruption of sedative infusions in critically ill patients undergoing mechanical ventilation. New England Journal of Medicine. 2000; 342(20): 1471-7.

9. Woods J, Mion L, Connor J, Viray F, Jahan L, Huber C, McHugh R, Gonzales J, Stoller J, Arroliga A. Severe agitation among ventilated medical intensive

care unit patients: Frequency, characteristics and outcomes. Intensive Care Med. 2004; 30(6):1066-72.

10. Vasile B, Rasulo F, Candiani A, Latronico N. The pathophysiology of propofol infusion syndrome: a simple name for a complex syndrome. Intensive Care Med. 2003; 29(9):1417-25.

11. Arroliga A, Shehab N, McCarthy K, Gonzales J. Relationship of continuous infusion lorazepam to serum propylene glycol concentration in critically ill adults. Critical Care Med. 2004; 32(8):1709-14.

12. Schweickert W, Gehlbach B, Pohlman A, Hall J, Kress J. Daily interruption of sedative infusions and complications of critical illness in mechanically ventilated patients. Critical Care Med. 2004; 32(6):1272-6.

13. Brook A, Ahrens T, Schaiff R, Prentice D, Sherman G, Shannon W, Kollef M. Effect of a nursing implemented sedation protocol on the duration of mechanical ventilation. Critical Care Med. 1999; 27(12): 2609-15.

14. Brattebo G, Hofoss D, Flaatten H, Muri A, Gjerde S, Plsek P. Effect of a scoring system and protocol for sedation on duration of patients' need for ventilator support in a surgical intensive care unit. BMJ. 2002; 324(7350):1386-9.

15. Pun B, Gordon S, Peterson J, Shintani A, Jackson J, Foss J, Harding S, Bernard G, Dittus R, Ely E. Large-scale implementation of sedation and delirium monitoring in the intensive care unit: A report from two medical centers. Critical Care Med. 2005; 33(6):1199-205.

16. Pronovost P, Berenholtz S, Dorman T, Lipsett P, Simmonds T, Haraden C. Improving communication in the ICU using daily goals. Journal of Critical Care. 2003; 18(2):71-5.

17. Grap M, Munro C, Wetzel P, Best A, Ketchum J, Hamilton V, Arief N, Pickler R, Sessler C. Sedation in adults receiving mechanical ventilation: Physiological and comfort outcomes. AACN. 2012; 21(3): 53-64

18. Walker N, Gillen P. Investigating nurses' perceptions of their role in managing sedation in intensive care: An exploratory study. Intensive and Critical Care Nursing. 2006; 22(6): 338–45.

19. Morgan R. Nurse training program: Current sedatives for intensive care setting. Anesthesiology News. 2007; 33(5): 2-21.

20. Ford S, Roach S. Roach's introductory clinical pharmacology. 9th ed. Philadelphia: Lippincott Williams & Wilkins. 2009; 18-24, 237-44.

21. Lewis M. Reliability study of the sedation-agitation scale in an intensive care unit. Victoria University of Wellington, Master thesis, 2004.

22. Carrasc G, Carbrel I. Sedation in intensive medicine. Intensive Care Med. 1999; 19(3):59-63.

23. Aitken L, Marshall A, Elliott R, McKinley S. Critical care nurses' decision making: Sedation assessment and management in intensive care. Journal of Clinical Nursing. 2009; 18(1):36-45.

24. Soliman H, Melit C, Vincent J. Sedation and analgesia practice in the intensive care unit: The result of European survey. BRJ Anaesth. 2001; 87(2):186-92.

25. Ba-alwi A. Impact of closed versus open tracheal suction on the occurrence of ventilator associated pneumonia. (Unpublished) Doctoral Thesis, Alexandria University, Faculty of Nursing, 2008.

26. Yagan M, White D, Staab J. Sedation of the mechanically ventilated patient. Critical Care Nurses. 2000; 22(4): 90–100.

27. Kress J, Pohlman A, Hall J. Sedation and analgesia in the intensive care unit. Respiratory and Critical Care Medicine. 2002; 166(8):1024-8.

28. Young C, Knudsen N, Hilton A, Reves J. Sedation in the intensive care unit. Critical Care Medicine. 2000; 28(3): 854-66.

29. Olson D. Combining observational and physiologic sedation assessment tools. University of North Carolina, Faculty of Nursing, 2007.

30. Rowe K, Fletcher S. Sedation in the intensive care unit. Continuing Education in Anesthesia, Critical Care & Pain journal. 2008; 8(2):50-5.

31. Dennis L, Mayer S. Diagnosis and management of increased intracranial pressure. Neurology India. 2001; 49 (1):37-50.

32. John P. Kress M, Jesse B. Hall M. Sedation in the mechanically ventilated patient. Critical Care Med. 2006; 1 (34):25-42.

33. Goodwin H, Lewin J, Mirski M. Cooperative sedation: optimizing comfort while maximizing systemic and neurological function. Critical Care. 2012; 16(2):1-7.

34. Chulay M, Burns S. AACN Essential of critical care nursing. 2ed ed. New York: McGraw-hill companies. 2010;163-76

35. Nasraway S, Jacobi J, Murray M, Lumb P, Task Force of the American College of Critical Care Medicine of the Society of Critical Care Medicine and the American Society of Health-System Pharmacists, American College of Chest Physicians. Sedation, analgesia, and neuromuscular blockade of the critically ill adult: Revised clinical practice guidelines for 2002. Critical Care Med. 2002; 30(1):117–8.

36. McCann M, Brustowicz R, Bacsik J, Sullivan L, Auble S, Laussen P. The bispectral index and explicit recall during the intra operative wake-up test for scoliosis surgery. Anesthesia and Analgesia.2002; 94(6):1474-8.

37. Burchardi H. Aims of sedation and analgesia. Minerva Anesthesiology. 2004; 70(4), 137-43.

38. Braun T, Hagen N, Clark T. Development of a clinical practice guideline for palliative sedation. Journal of Palliative Medicine. 2003; 6(3): 345-50.

39. Muller H, Andres I, Jehser T. Sedation in palliative care: A critical analysis of 7 years experience. BMC Palliative Care. 2003; 2(1): 2.

40. American Society of Anesthesiologists. Continuum of depth of sedation: Definitions of general anesthesia and levels of sedation/analgesia. 2009. Available at: http://www.asahq.org/Home/For-Members/Clinical-Information/Standards-Guidelines-and-Statements. Retrieved on: 23/4/2012.

41.   Garber A, Webster B. Clinical procedure: Adult procedural sedation. Swedish Health Services. 2010. Available at: http://www.swedish.org/Search/Results?utility_search=Clinical+procedure%3A+adult+procedural+sedation#axzz22Wo3r0Bi. Retrieved on: 30/3/2012.

42.   American Society of Anesthesiologists (ASA). Practice guidelines for sedation/analgesia by none anesthesiologists. 2001. available at: http://www.asahq.org/publications_and_services/sedation1017.pdf. Retrieved on: 12/4/2012.

43.   Rowe K, Fletcher S. Sedation in the intensive care unit. Continuing Education in Anesthesia, Critical Care and Pain. 2008; 8(2):50-5.

44.   Short J. Use of dexmedetomidine for primary sedation in a general intensive care unit. Critical Care Nurse. 2010; 30(1): 29-38.

45.   Magarey J. Sedation of adult critically ill ventilated patients in intensive care units: A national survey. Australian Critical Care Nurses. 1997; 10(3): 90-3.

46.   Tung A, Tadimeti L, Caruana B, Atkins P, Mion L, Palmer R, Slomka J, Mendelson W. The relationship of sedation to deliberate self-extubation. Journal of Clinical Anesthesia. 2001; 13(1): 24-9.

47.   Olson D, Chioffi S, Macy G, Meek L, Cook H. Potential benefits of bispectral index monitoring in critical care. Critical Care Nurse. 2003; 23(4): 45-52.

48.   Rinaldi S, Consales G, De Gaudio A. Sedation monitoring in ICU. Current Anesthesia & Critical Care. 2006; 17(5): 303–15

49.   Sessler C, Varney K. Patient-focused sedation and analgesia in the ICU. American college of chest physicians. 2008; 133(2):552-65.

50.   Sessler C, Grap M, Brophy G. Multidisciplinary management of sedation and analgesia in critical care. *Respiratory* Critical *Care Med*. 2001; 22(2):211-26.

51.   Ostermann M, Keenan S, Seiferling R, Sibbald W. Sedation in the intensive care unit: A systematic review. JAMA. 2000; 283(11):1451-9.

52. Ashton H. Benzodiazepines: How they work and how to withdraw. The Ashton Manual. 2002. Available at: http://benzo.org.uk/ annual/index.htm. Retrieved on: 22/5/2012.

53. Young C, Prielipp R. Benzodiazepines in the intensive care unit. Critical Care Clin. 2001; 17(4):843-62.

54. Urden L, Stacy K, Lough M. Critical care nursing diagnosis and management. 5th ed. New York: Mosby Inc. 2006; 220-5.

55. Deglin J, Vallerand A, Sanoski C. Davis's drug guide for nurses. 12th ed. Philadelphia: Davis Company. 2011; 431-4, 859-61, 1066-8.

56. Papadakos P. Approach to sedation and airway management in the ICU in Apostolakos M. The intensive care manual. New York: McGraw-Hill. 2001; 350-4.

57. Turan I, Sahin C. Paradoxic reaction to midazolam during intravenous sedation. Journal of Anesthesiology. 2008; 16 (1):15.

58. Dipiro J, Talbert R, Yee G, Matzke G, Wells B, Posey M. Pharmacotherapy: A pathophysiologic approach. 6th ed. New York: McGraw-Hill. 2005; 1321-33.

59. Rhoney D, Parker D. Use of sedative and analgesic agents in neurotrauma patients: Effects on cerebral physiology. Neurological Research. 2001; 23(3): 237-59.

60. Weekes L, Gillis J. Sedation of the intensive care patient. 1995. Available at: http://www.nsw.gov.au/search/search?simulate_xml_version=9.0.x&cluster0 =sedation+of+the+intensive+care+patient+1995&remote_ip=41.129.69.207& query=sedation+of+the+intensive+care+patient+1995+|u%3ahealth.nsw.gov. au. Retrieved on: 15/3/2012.

61. Evers A, Crowder C. General anesthetics. In: Hardman J, Limbird L. Goodman and Gilman's The pharmacological basis of therapeutics, 10th ed. New York: McGraw-Hill. 2001; 337–65.

62. Mirski M, Hemstreet M. Critical care sedation for neuroscience patients. Journal of the Neurological Sciences. 2007; 261(1):16-34

63. Lacy C, Armstrong L, Goldman M, Lance L. Drug information handbook. 18th ed. New York: Lexi-Comp. 2010; 1170-9.

64. Angelini G, Ketzler J, Coursin D. Use of propofol and other non-benzodiazepine sedatives in the intensive care unit. Critical Care Clin. 2001; 17(4):863-80.

65. Whitcomb J, Huddleston M, McAndrews K. The use of propofol in the mechanically ventilated medical/surgical intensive care patient: Is it the right choice. Critical Care Nurse. 2003; 22(2):60-3.

66. Morton P, Fontaine D. Critical care nursing: A holistic approach. 9th ed. Philadelphia: Lippincott Williams & Wilkins. 2009; 866-9.

67. Mirski M, Muffelman B, Ulatowski J, Hanely D. Sedation for the critically ill neurologic patient. Critical Care Medicine. 1995; 23(12): 2038-53.

68. Clayton B, Stock Y, Harroun R. Basic pharmacology for nurses. 14th ed. Paris: Mosby Inc. 2007; 383-4.

69. Marino P. The ICU book. 3th ed. New York: Lippincott Williams & Wilkins. 2007; 947-58

70. Alexander E, Lam S, Sulsa G. Drug update: Dexmedetomidine use in critical care. AACN. 2008;19(2):113-20

71. Sackey P, Martling C, Carlsward C, Sundin O, Radell P. Short- and long-term follow-up of intensive care unit patients after sedation with isoflurane and midazolam: A pilot study. Critical Care Med. 2008; 36(3):801–6

72. Sackey P, Martling C, Granath F, Radell P. Prolonged isoflurane sedation of intensive care unit patients with the anesthetic conserving device. Critical Care Medicine. 2004; 32(11):2241–6

73. Gommers D, Bakker J. Medications for analgesia and sedation in the intensive care unit: An overview. Critical Care. 2008; 3 (12):S4.

74. Wagner B, O'Hara D. Pharmacokinetics and pharmacodynamics of sedatives and analgesics in the treatment of agitated and critically ill patients. Clinical pharmacokinetic. 1997; 33(6): 426-53

75.   Kumar P. Sedation and pain relief. Indian Journal of Anesthesia. 2003; 47(5): 396-401.

76.   Belda E, Sora M, Meiser A. Sedation with inhaled anesthetics in intensive care. In   Vincent J. Intensive Care Medicine: Annual update. New York: Springer Berlin Heidelberg. 2008; 839-49.

77.   Peck M, Down J. Use of sedatives in the critically ill. Anesthesia and Intensive Care Medicine. 2010; 11(1): 12-5.

78.   White S, Hollet J, Kress J, Zellinger M. A renaissance in critical care nursing: Technological advances and sedation strategies. Critical Care Nurse. 2001; 21(5): 1-14.

79.   Girard T, Kress J, Fuchs B, Thomason J, Schweickert W, Pun B, Taichman D, Dunn J, Pohlman A, Kinniry P, Jackson J, Canonico A, Light R, Shintani A, Thompson J, Gordon S, Hall J, Dittus R, Bernard G, Ely E. Efficacy and safety of a paired sedation and ventilator weaning protocol for mechanically ventilated patients in intensive care (awakening and breathing controlled trial): A randomized controlled trial. Lancet. 2008; 371(9607):126–34.

80.   Kress J. Daily interruption of sedation in mechanically ventilated patients: The ICU sedation vacation. 6th conference sedation therapy. 2005. Available at: https://docs.google.com/viewer?a=v&q=cache:6kigT2QRekwJ:www.premier inc.com/safety/topics/patient_safety/downloads/sedation-proceedings.pdf. Retrieved on: 23/4/2012.

81.   Ramsay M. The role of brain monitoring in the ICU. 6th conference sedation therapy.   2005.   Available   at: https://docs.google.com/viewer?a=v&q=cache:6kigT2QRekwJ:www.premier inc.com/safety/topics/patient_safety/downloads/sedation-proceedings.pdf. Retrieved on: 23/4/2012.

82.   Devlin J, Boleski G, Mlynarek M, Nerenz D, Peterson E, Jankowski M, Horst H, Zarowitz B. Motor Activity Assessment Scale: A valid and reliable sedation scale for use with mechanically ventilated patients in an adult surgical intensive care unit. Critical Care Medicine.1999; 27(7):1271-5.

83.   Diawai O, Thoyre S, Auyong D. Perspectives on sedation assessment in critical care. Advanced Critical Care. 2007; 18(4): 380-95.

84.   Rassin M, Sruyah R, Kahalon A, Naveh R, Nicar I, Silner D. Between the fixed and changing: Examining and comparing reliability and validity of 3 sedation-agitation measuring scales. Dimensions of Critical Care Nursing. 2007; 26(2): 76-82.

85.   Ely W, Truman B, Shintani A, Thomason J, Wheeler A, Gordon S, Francis J, Speroff T, Gautam S, Margolin R, Sessler C, Dittus R, Bernard G. Monitoring sedation status over time in ICU patients. Intensive Care medicine. 2003; 289(22):2983-91.

86.   Jullette A. Analysis of sedation scales in assessing sedation levels of the traumatic brain injured patient. Master thesis. University of Arizona, Faculty of Nursing, 2010.

87.   Simmons L, Riker R, Prato B, Fraser G. Assessing sedation during intensive care unit mechanical ventilation with the bispectral index and the Sedation-Agitation Scale. Critical Care Medicine. 1999; 27(8):1499-504.

88.   Aspect Medical Systems. Company information. Available at: Http://www.aspectmscom. Retrieved on: 11/5/2012.

89.   Holtzhausen R. Principles and process of critical care nursing. 2011. Available at: http://www.scribd.com/doc/58578521/Principles-and-Process-of-Critical-Care-Nursing-60143-742-Best-Practice-Sedation-Rudi-Holtzhausen-15238849. Retrieved on: 25/5/2012.

90.   Institute for Safe Medication Practices (ISMP's). Available at: http://www.ismp.org/. Retrieved on: 28/6/2012.

91.   Hardmeier B, Braunschweig S, Cavallaro M, Roos M, Pauli C, Giger M, Meier P, Fattinger K. Adverse drug events caused by medication errors in medical inpatients. Swiss Medical Weekly. 2004; 134(46): 664-70.

92.   Pepper G. "Errors in drug administration by nurses." American Journal of Health-System Pharmacy. 1995; 52 (4): 390-5.

93.   Smith J. Building safer NHS for patients: Improving medication safety. Department of Health. 2004. Available at: http://www.doh.gov.uk/buildsafenhs/medicationsafety. Retrieved on: 1/5/2012.

94.   Schull D. Five rights still resound. Nurse Week (South Central). 2005; 12(20): 9 - 18.

95.   Rich D. "New JCAHO medication management standards for 2004." American Journal of Health-System Pharmacy. 2004; 61(13): 1349-58.

96.   Mansour M. Critical care nurses' views on medication administration: An organizational perspective. Doctoral thesis. University of Nottingham, Faculty of Nursing, 2009.

97.   Egerod I. Uncertain terms of sedation in ICU: How nurse and physicians manage and describe sedation for mechanically ventilated patients. Journal of Clinical Nursing. 2002; 11(6):831-40.

98.   Slomka J, Hoffman L, Mion L, Bair N, Bobek M, Arroliga A. Influence of clinician's values and perceptions on use of clinical practice guidelines for sedation. American Association of Critical Care Nurses. 2000; 9(6):412-8.

99.   Medication Administration: Guidelines for registered nurses. Saskatchewan Registered Nurses' Association (SRNA). 2007. Available at: http://www.srna.o...medication_admin.pdf. Retrieved on: 9/5/2012.

100. Kienle P, John P. Maintaining Compliance with Joint Commission Medication Management Standards. Patient safety & quality health care. 2008. Available at: http://www.psqh.com/julaug08/medication.html. Retrieved on: 13/3/2012.

101. Guidelines on sedation for procedures. Royal North Shore Hospital. Intensive Care Manual. 2006. Available at: http://www.directory.nsw.gov.au/search.asp?q=Guidelines%20on%20sedatio n%20for%20procedures&cx=018237954339939719400:_jbwc6fxs54&cof=F ORID%3A11&S=Directory. Retrieved on:3/3/2012

102.   Pun B, Dunn J. The sedation of critically ill adults (Part 2): Management. The American Journal of Nursing. 2007; 107(8): 40-9.

103. Implementing and ensuring safe sedation practice for healthcare procedures in adults. The Royal College of Anesthetists. 2001. Available at: http://www.rcoa.ac.uk/node/2270. Retrieved on: 15/5/2012.

104. Woodrow P. Intensive care nursing: A framework for practice. 2ed ed. New York: Taylor and Francis Group. 2006; 60-7.

105. Sweetman S. Martindale: The complete drug reference. 36th ed. London: Pharmaceutical Press. 2009; 992-3, 1792.

106. Standards and intents for sedation and analgesia care. Joint Commission on Accreditation of HealthCare Organizations (JCAHO). 2000. Available at: http://www.jointcommission.org/. Retrieved on: 28/4/2012.

107. Werrett G. Sedation in intensive care patients. Update in Anesthesia. 2003. Available at: http://www.nda.ox.ac.uk/wfsa/html/u16/u1605_01.htm. Retrieved on: 12/4/2012.

108. Schull P. Nursing spectrum drug handbook. 5th ed. New York: McGraw-Hill Companies. 2010; 339-40,684

109. McEvoy G, Bethesda M. AHFS drug information. American Society of Hospital Pharmacists. 2004. Available at: http://www.drugs.com/monograph/diazepam.html. Retrieved on: 28/5/2012.

110. Medication guidelines for registered nurses. College of registered nurses of Nova Scotia. 2011. Available at: http://www.crnns.ca/default.asp?id=190&sfield=content.id&search=4423&mn=414.1116.1130.2384.2389. Retrieved on:13/6/2012

111. Pharmacy and therapeutics committee. Use of minimal sedation for clinic appointments and diagnostic procedures. 2004. Available at: www.centralstatehospital.org/policy/Policy4.54.pdf. Retrieved on: 12/3/2012.

112. Olson D, Graffagnino C, King K, Lynch J. Toward solving the sedation-assessment conundrum: Bispectral index monitoring and sedation interruption. Critical Care Nursing Clinics North America. 2005; 17(3): 257-67.

113. Bradley A. Clinical pharmacology of sedatives in the critically ill. 6th conference sedation therapy. 2005. Available at: https://docs.google.com/viewer?a=v&q=cache:6kigT2QRekwJ:www.premier inc.com/safety/topics/patient_safety/downloads/sedation-proceedings.pdf. Retrieved on: 23/4/2012.

114. Mills E. Nursing procedures. 4th ed. Virginia: Lippincott Williams & Wilkins. 2004; 229-32, 242-4, 248-53.

115. Rhoads J, Meeker B. Davis's guide to clinical nursing skills. 10th ed. Philadelphia: Davis Company. 2008; 155-83.

116. Temple J, Johnson J. Nurses' guide to clinical procedures. 5th ed. New York: Lippincott Williams & Wilkins. 2006; 279-94.

117. Abrams A. Clinical drug therapy: Rationales for nursing practice. 7th ed. Lippincott Williams & Wilkins. 2003; 43-5.

118. Guttormsona J, Chlana L, Weinertb C, Savik K. Factors influencing nurse sedation practices with mechanically ventilated patients: A U.S. national survey. Intensive and Critical Care Nursing. 2010; 26 (1): 44-50

119. El Shenawi S. Establishing standard for prevention and control of nosocomial infection in the intensive care units at the Alexandria main university hospital. (Unpublished) Doctoral Thesis, Alexandria University, Faculty of Nursing, 2002.

120. Mehta S, Maureen O, Hynes P, Woganee A, Burry L, Hallett D. A multicenter survey of Ontario intensive care unit nurses regarding the use of sedatives and analgesics for adults receiving mechanical ventilation. Journal of Critical Care. 2007; 22 (3): 191–6

121. O'Connor M, Bucknall T, Manias E. Sedation management in Australian and New Zealand ICUs: Doctors and nurses practice and opinions. American Association of Critical Care Nurses. 2010; 19 (3):285-95.

122. Martin J, Franck M, Sigel S, Weiss M, Spies C. Changes in sedation management in German intensive care units between 2002 and 2006: A national follow up survey. Crit Care 2007; 11(6): 1-7.

123. Tanios M, Marjolein D, Scott K, John W. Perceived barriers to the use of sedation protocols and daily sedation interruption: A multidisciplinary survey. Journal of Critical Care. 2009; 24 (1): 66–73.

124. Reschreiter H, Maiden M, Kapila A. Sedation practice in the intensive care unit: A UK national survey. Critical Care. 2008; 12(6): 1-8.

125. Weir S, Neill A. Experiences of intensive care nurses assessing sedation/agitation in critically ill patients. British Association of Critical Care Nurses, Nursing in Critical Care. 2008; 13(4):185-94.

126. De Jonghe B, Bastuji-Garin S, Fangio P, Lacherade J, Jabot J, Rocha N, Outin H. Sedation algorithm in critically ill patients without acute brain injury. Critical Care Medicine. 2005; 33 (1):120-7.

127. Samuelson K, Larsson S, Lundberg D, Fridlund B. Intensive care sedation of mechanically ventilated patients: A national Swedish survey. Intensive and Critical Care Nursing. 2003; 19 (6):350–62.

128. Randen I, Bjørk I. Sedation practice in three Norwegian ICUs: A survey of intensive care nurses' perceptions of personal and unit practice. Intensive and Critical Care Nursing. 2010; 26 (5): 270-7.

129. Joanna H. Sedation in mechanically ventilated patients. Highline Medical Center. 2009; 30(2):1-2.

130. Wunsch H, Kress J. A New Era for Sedation in ICU Patients. JAMA. 2009; 301(5): 544.

131. Murdoch S, Cohen A. Intensive care sedation: A review of current British practice. Intensive Care Medicine. 2000; 26(6): 922–8.

132. El Sayed M. Nurses' medication administration practices and sources of errors. (Unpublished) Master Thesis, Alexandria University, Faculty of Nursing, 2012.

133. Weinert C, Chlan L, Gross C. Sedating critically ill patients: Factors affecting nurses' delivery of sedative therapy. AACN. 2001; 10(3): 156-65.

134. Beyea S, Hicks R. The patient is allergic to that medication: Patient safety first. The Association of perioperative registered nurses (AORN). 2003. Available

at: http://www.highbeam.com/doc/1G1-99237614.html. Retrieved on: 25/6/2012.

135. Gaber M. Nurses' perception and satisfaction towards caregivers' collaboration in intensive care units. (Unpublished) Master Thesis, Alexandria University, Faculty of Nursing, 2010.

136. Westcott C. The sedation of patients' intensive care units: A nursing review. Intensive and Critical Care Nursing. 1995; 11(1):26-31

137. Miller K. Early awakening and sedation reduction. Respiratory Care. 2010. available at: http://www.rtmagazine.com/issues/articles/2010-11_03.asp. Retrieved on 26/7/2012.

138. Salgado D, Brimioulle S. Toward less sedation in the intensive care unit: A prospective observational study. Journal of Critical Care. 2010; 26(2):113-21.

139. Aboud R. Mechanically ventilated patients' communication needs. (Unpublished) Master Thesis, Alexandria University, Faculty of Nursing, 2008.

140. Ramsay M. Measuring level of sedation in the intensive care unit. JAMA. 2000; 284(4):441–2.

141. Abd El-Razak M. The usefulness of pain assessment and intervention notation tool in critical care nursing practice. (Unpublished) Master Thesis, Alexandria University, Faculty of Nursing, 2005.

142. Kathleen S, Tracey B. Pain assessment in critical care: What have we learnt from research?. Intensive and Critical Care Nursing. 2003; 19 (3):154-62.

143. Sharkawy F, Reda N, Attia A, Ibrahim Y. Pain as a fifth vital sign in a standardized pain flow sheet: Impact on patient-reported pain experience after cardiovascular surgery. AJAIC. 2004:7(1): 26-34.

144. Jackson D, Proudfoot C, Cann K, Walsh T. A systematic review of the impact of sedation practice in the ICU on resource use, costs and patient safety. Critical Care. 2010; 14(2):9-10.

الملخص العربي

الملخص العربي

تستخدم الأدوية المهدئة بشكل كبير في وحدات العناية الحرجة ويعتبر إعطاؤها جزءً أساسياً من الرعاية المقدمة لمرضى العناية الحرجة. حيث أن هؤلاء المرضى في معظم الأحيان يكونون على جهاز التنفس الإصطناعي ويعانون من أمراض خطيرة ويخضعون بإستمرار لإجراءات علاجية وتشخيصية. يهدف إعطاء الأدوية المهدئة بشكل أساسي إلى زيادة شعور المريض بالراحة ومنعه من أذية نفسه وزيادة تقبله لجهاز التنفس الإصطناعي، تقليل الإجهاد البدني والنفسي وتسهيل تحمل المريض للإجراءات العلاجية والتشخيصية التي يخضع لها، بالإضافة إلى أهداف علاجية أخرى مثل خفض الضغط داخل الدماغ عند المرضى المصابين بإصابات الرأس أوالسكتة الدماغية.

إن الأدوية المهدئة، بما تمتلكه من خصائص وباعتبارها من الأدوية ذات الخطورة العالية، تحتاج إلى إنتباه وحذر شديد في التعامل معها حيث أن الإستخدام الخاطئ والعشوائي لها يؤدي إلى مضاعفات كثيرة وخطيرة على حياة المرضى في وحدات العناية الحرجة. ولتحقيق الإستخدام الأمثل لهذه الأدوية يجب أن يتم إعطاؤها بناء على بروتوكول خاص بالأدوية المهدئة يتم تطويره وتعديله حسب نوعية مرضى وحدات العناية الحرجة، بالإضافة إلى إستخدام مقياس تهدئة sedation scale للحفاظ على مستوى معين من التهدئة sedation level لكل مريض على حسب حالته بحيث لا يزيد أو ينقص عن المستوى المطلوب،حيث أن هذه الزيادة أو النقصان ،أو ما يسمى بفرط التهدئة ونقص التهدئة، كل منها له مضاعفات خطيرة على حياة المريض.

يلعب الكادر التمريضي دوراً محورياً وهاماً في إعطاء الأدوية المهدئة باعتباره جزءً أساسياً من مسؤولياته. إذ أن الممرض من خلال متابعته للمريض على مدار اليوم قادر على القيام بتقييم مستمر لمستوى التهدئة عند المريض وإكتشاف أي إنحراف عن المستوى المطلوب سواء بالزيادة أو بالنقصان، بالإضافة إلى أنه قادر على إعطاء معلومات مهمة عن فعالية الدواء المهدئ المستخدم ومدى تحقيقه للهدف المطلوب. يجب على ممرضي العناية الحرجة الذين يقومون بإعطاء الأدوية المهدئة أن يمتلكوا معلومات كافية عن الدواء من ناحية تأثيره ومدة عمله و الأثار الجانبية المتوقعة والإحتياطات الخاصة بإعطاء كل دواء بالإضافة إلى معلومات كافية عن دورهم قي تقييم المريض قبل وأثناء وبعد إعطاء الأدوية المهدئة ومراقبة التأثيرات المتوقعة وغير المتوقعة وكيفية التصرف في حال حدوث مضاعفات.

ويجب عليهم ترجمة هذه المعلومات التي يمتلكونها عمليًا أثناء إعطاء الأدوية المهدئة لتحقيق الإستخدام الأمثل والآمن لهذه الأدوية.

هدف الدراسة: تهدف هذه الدراسة إلى تحديد مستوى المعلومات والممارسات لدى ممرضي العناية الحرجة فيما يتعلق بالإستخدام الآمن للأدوية المهدئة.

أدوات وطرق البحث:

مكان الدراسة: تم إجراء هذه الدراسة في وحدة عناية الحوادث (الوحدة الأولى) ووحدة العناية العامة (الوحدة الثالثة) والتي تنتمي إلى وحدات العناية الحرجة بالمستشفى الرئيسي الجامعي بالإسكندرية.

عينة الدراسة: شملت عينة الدراسة خمسين ممرض وممرضة في وحدتي العناية الحرجة المذكورة أعلاه.

أدوات الدراسة:

تم جمع بيانات الدراسة عن طريق أداتي بحث قام الباحث بتصميمهما بعد إستعراض شامل للمراجع ذات الصلة(4, 34, 55, 68, 90, 96, 110, 114-117).

- **الأداة الأولى:** **"ممارسات ممرضي العناية الحرجة المتعلقه بالإستخدام الآمن للأدوية المهدئة":** وهي عبارة عن قائمة تدقيق ملاحظاتية لقياس أداء ممرضي العناية الحرجة فيما يتعلق بإعطاء الأدوية المهدئة.

- **الأداة الثانية:** **"معلومات ممرضي العناية الحرجة المتعلقة بالإستخدام الآمن للأدوية المهدئة":** وهي عبارة عن إستبيان لقياس مستوى المعرفة والمعلومات عن الأدوية المهدئة لدى ممرضي العناية الحرجة.

منهج الدراسة :

- تمّ الحصول على الموافقة لإجراء الدراسة من الجهات المعنية في المستشفى الرئيسي الجامعي في مدينة الإسكندرية بعد تقديم شرح كافٍ عن الهدف من إجراء هذه الدراسة.

- قام الباحث بتطوير أداتي البحث بعد إستعراض شامل للمراجع ذات الصلة.

- تمّ إختبار مصداقية المحتوى من خلال عرض أداتي الدراسة على سبع خبراء، أربعة منهم أساتذة من أعضاء هيئة التدريس في مجال تمريض العناية الحرجة والطوارىء في كلية التمريض بجامعة الإسكندرية، وثلاثة أساتذة في مجال طب الأدوية في كلية الصيدلة بجامعة الإسكندرية، وتمّ إجراء التعديلات اللازمة وفقًا لذلك.

- تمّ الحصول على موافقة شفهية من كل ممرض/ة على حدا للمشاركة في الدراسة وذلك بعد شرح الهدف من إجرائها. وتمّ إبلاغ المشاركين في الدراسة بأن المشاركة طوعية وأنه يحق لأي ممرض/ة الإنسحاب من الدراسة في أي وقت ولا يترتب على ذلك أي مسؤولية.

- تمّ إجراء دراسة تجريبية مصغرة على عشر ممرضات/ين للتأكد من وضوح أدوات البحث ومن قابليتها للتطبيق العملي، وتم إستبعاد المشاركين فيها من العدد الإجمالي لعينة الدراسة.

- تمّ التحقق من ثبات أداة الدراسة الثانية "معلومات ممرضي العناية الحرجة المتعلقة بالإستخدام الآمن للأدوية المهدئة" عن طريق إجراء إختبار معامل كرونباخ ألفا / Cronbach`s coefficient alpha / وكانت النتيجة مقبوله (0.72 = r).

- تمّ جمع البيانات المطلوبة عن طريق أداتي الدراسة كما يلي:

• الملاحظة: استخدمت فيها الأداة الأولى لتقييم أداء الممرضات أثناء إعطاء الأدوية المهدئة. تم ملاحظة أداء كل ممرض/ة ثلاث مرات أثناء إعطاء الأدوية المهدئة خلال ثلاث ورديات مختلفة (صباحاً، مساءً، ليلا).

• الإستبيان: بعد الإنتهاء من جميع الملاحظات تم توزيع الإستبيانات على الممرضات/ين الذين تم ملاحظتهم سابقاً. ويهدف هذا الإستبيان إلى تقييم معلومات الممرضات/ين المتعلقة بالأدوية المهدئة. وتمت الإجابة على الإستبيان من قبل الممرض/ة خلال الوردية (النوبتجية) وأثناء وجود الباحث ثم تم جمع الإستبيانات من قبل الباحث مع نهاية الوردية (النوبتجية).

- تم جمع البيانات خلال فترةٍ زمنيةٍ إمتدت لثلاث شهور مابين (10-1- 2012) إلى (5-4- 2012) .

- تمّ إجراء التحليل الإحصائي للبيانات حاسوبياً بإستخدام الإصدار السادس عشر من برنامج التحليل الإحصائي (SPSS).

النتائج الرئيسية للدراسة:

- أظهرت نتائج الدراسة أن معظم أعمار المشاركين فيها أقل من 25 سنة و أن أكثر من نصف عينة الدراسة كان من الإناث. أما بالنسبة لمستوى التعلُّم فقد كان أكثر من ثلاثة أرباع العينة من خريجي كلية التمريض والباقي من خريجي المعهد الفني التمريضي. أكثر من نصف العينة كانوا يعملون في وحدة عناية الحوادث (الوحدة الأولى). حوالي ثلثي العينة كان لديهم خبرة في وحدات العناية الحرجة لأقل من سنة.

116

- كما أظهرت نتائج الدراسة الحالية أن مستوى المعلومات لدى ممرضي العناية الحرجة فيما يتعلق بالأدوية المهدئة عموماً متوسط. أما مستوى الممارسة لدى ممرضي العناية الحرجة فيما يتعلق بالأدوية المهدئة فهو ضعيف.

- جميع ممرضي العناية الحرجة لا يستخدمون مقياس تهدئة، كما أنه لا يوجد بروتوكول خاص بالأدوية المهدئة ينظم طريقة إعطائها بالإضافة إلى عدم وجود تعاون وتنسيق بين الكادر الطبي والتمريضي فيما يتعلق بتحديد مستوى التهدئة لدى مرضى العناية الحرجة.

- هناك علاقة ذات أهمية إحصائية بين مستوى المعلومات لدى ممرضي العناية الحرجة وبين الخبرة، حيث أن الممرضين الذين لديهم سنوات خبرة أكثر في مجال تمريض العناية الحرجة مستوى المعلومات لديهم أفضل من الممرضين الأقل خبرة (المتوسط الحسابي = 55.2±9.2).

- الأدوية المهدئة الأكثر إستخداماً في وحدات العناية الحرجة التي أجريت فيها الدراسة هي (بروبوفول، ميدازولام وديازيبام). كما أظهرت نتائج الدراسة أن أكثر دواعي إستعمال الأدوية المهدئة هي لتقليل القلق والهيجان لدى مرضى العناية الحرجة وتسهيل تحملهم لجهاز التنفس الإصطناعي .

- أظهرت نتائج الدراسة أن مستوى التهدئة لدى مرضى العناية الحرجة كان مناسباً لحوالي النصف منهم. أما الباقون فكان مستوى التهدئة عندهم غير مناسب لحالتهم حيث كان لديهم إما فرط تهدئة أو نقص تهدئة.

التوصيات المقترحة:

1- يجب أن تتضمن مناهج التدريس في كليات التمريض والمعاهد والمدارس المتخصصة معلومات كافية حول الأدوية المهدئة مع زيادة التركيز على تدريب الطلاب على طرق تقييم مستوى التهدئة.

2- تنظيم مؤتمرات وبرامج توعية قبل التوظيف بكل ما يتعلق بالأدوية المهدئة بالإضافة إلى برامج تعليمية وتدريبية للكادر التمريضي بشكل دوري و التي من شأنها رفع مستوى المعرفة والوعي لدى ممرضي العناية الحرجة عن أهمية الأدوية المهدئة وطرق الإستخدام الأمثل لها.

3- يجب أن تتوافر في المشافي ووحدات العناية الحرجة كل الإمكانيات التي من شأنها تسهيل وصول الكادر التمريضي للمعلومات التي يحتاجها بما في ذلك المجلات والكتب العلمية الحديثة و نتائج الأبحاث المحلية والعالمية, بالإضافة إلى إرشادات وتوجيهات خاصة بالأدوية المهدئة مكتوبة ومتاحة في مختلف وحدات العناية الحرجة.

4- تطوير السياسات المتعلقة بإعطاء الأدوية المهدئة وذلك من خلال إدخال بروتوكول أو دليل ينظم ويضبط آلية التعامل مع الأدوية المهدئة و المرضى الذين يعالجون بها.

5- العمل على توفير مكتبة علمية ضمن المستشفى تكون متاحة للكادر الطبي والتمريضي ومزودة بأحدث الكتب والأبحاث العلمية مع سهولة الوصول إلى المعلومات عن طريق الإنترنت.

6- العمل على إدخال مقاييس التهدئة بأنواعها إلى الممارسة العملية وتدريب الكادر التمريضي على كيفية إستخدامها.

7- تقييم مستوى التهدئة لدى مرضى العناية الحرجة بشكل منتظم.

8- توعية الكادر التمريضي بأهمية دورهم أثناء إستخدام الأدوية المهدئة وضرورة مشاركتهم للكادر الطبي في عملية إتخاذ القرار الخاص بمستوى التهدئة لدى كل مريض.

9- إستخدام بروتوكول أو دليل معتمد ينظم إستخدام الأدوية المهدئة في وحدات العناية الحرجة.

10- حث الكادر الطبي ومشرفي التمريض على المتابعة الدائمة لممرضي العناية الحرجة لمستوى التهدئة من خلال توجيه الأسئلة بإستمرار لمقدمي الرعاية التمريضية عن مستوى التهدئة لدى مرضاهم.

11- إعادة تصميم سجلات التمريض بإضافة جزء خاص حول مقياس التهدئة وتوعية الكادر التمريضي لضرورة التعامل معه على أساس أنه سادس العلامات الحيوية.

12- العمل على تأمين الأدوات الضرورية والتي تساعد على تقييم مستوى التهدئة وبشكل خاص جهاز (bispectral index monitor) ليكون متاحاً في كل وحدات العناية الحرجة.

13- إجراء المزيد من الأبحاث وعلى مستوى أوسع وأشمل تتناول الأدوية المهدئة من نواحي أخرى مثل:

- تأثير الإيقاف التدريجي للأدوية المهدئة على فترة بقاء المريض على جهاز التنفس الإصطناعي.

- العوامل المؤثرة على ممارسات ممرضي العناية الحرجة المتعلقة بالأدوية المهدئة.

- تأثير إستخدام بروتوكول ومقياس التهدئة على المضاعفات المتعلقة بالأدوية المهدئة.

- تأثير إستخدام جهاز (bispectral index monitor) في تحديد مستوى التهدئة لدى مرضى العناية الحرجة.

- إعادة هذه الدراسة على عينة أكبر للتمكن من تعميم النتائج على نطاق أوسع.

www.ingramcontent.com/pod-product-compliance
Lightning Source LLC
Chambersburg PA
CBHW070408200326
41518CB00011B/2114